Intermittent Fasting

The Real Secret to Weight Loss & Living Healthy

Fitness & Health Fuel

advice. The content of this book has been derived from various sources. Please consult a licensed professional before attempting any techniques outlined in this book.

By reading this document, the reader agrees that under no circumstances are is the author responsible for any losses, direct or indirect, which are incurred as a result of the use of information contained within this document, including, but not limited to, —errors, omissions, or inaccuracies.

WAIT! Sign Up Now And

Get A FREE Bonus!

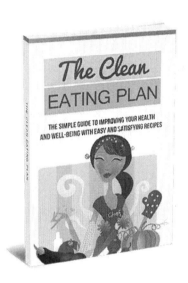

Discover How To Finally Take Control Of Your Diet And Eat Cleaner

- Discover how to eat healthier and cleaner without extra effort

- How your body works and how you can lose weight

- **How to train yourself so that you can eat cleaner forever**

- How to set and achieve your short and long term health goals

- **How to minimize time spent preparing meals**

- And so much more...

https://dibblypublishing.com/fht-bonuses

Contents

Introduction

Intermittent fasting has been in existence since time - immemorial. In fact, it spans the history of mankind. The regular 3-4 meals a day that we eat today is an anomaly in human evolution. Let us go into the history of eating patterns of our ancestors to understand this anomaly a little better. Our predecessors had certain feeding patterns that we have implanted into the modern world, and before we fully understand the concept of intermittent fasting, we're going to first look into the past.

Breakfast

For large parts of history, the concept of breakfast did not even exist. The Romans did not know what breakfast was. They ate one big meal around noon every day because they believed that eating once a day was a healthy option, and consuming more than one meal was frowned upon as gluttony. The Romans took their digestive system very seriously and ensured it was not unnecessarily stressed, except for sufficient nourishing of the body which they believed was fulfilled by eating just one full meal a day around noon.

The monastic way of life dictated eating patterns during the Middle Ages. No food was allowed before morning mass, and meats were restricted on many days of the year. Food historians opine that meat was not allowed to be consumed on nearly half the days of the year during the Middle Ages.

It appears that the concept of 'breakfast' was introduced into the English language around this time, and literally meant 'a meal to break the night's fast.' The English breakfast concept of bacon and eggs also seems to have originated from religion during the Middle Ages.

The Monday and Tuesday before Ash Wednesday, and the beginning of the Lent period, a specified timeframe where abstinence from meat is practiced, people had to exhaust their meat reserves which were typically pork and bacon. The meat was eaten with eggs which also needed to be used up before Lent began. And thus, was born the precursor to bacon and eggs! However, this dish was not eaten in the mornings. It was eaten around noon, as the people were accustomed to.

It was during the 17th century that the high-class society started consuming meals in the morning, or breakfast. The wealthy people began their day with scrambled eggs, coffee, and tea. By about 1740s, the rich class started having separate breakfast rooms in their homes. By the 19th century, new levels of breakfast decadence were reached, and plenty of dishes (historians put this number at 24!) were served in the morning.

The Industrial Revolution of the 19th century brought about standardization of work timings for industrial workers, and they needed something substantial in the morning to sustain them throughout the working day. Everyone began eating breakfast as part of their daily routines; from workers who spent their day fulfilling their duties, and even their bosses who only tend to sit around, supervising.

At the beginning of the 20th century, John Harvey Kellogg, the creator of cornflakes, revolutionized the concept of breakfast by turning it into a multi-billion dollar industry, marking how breakfast has evolved to the way it now stands today.

Breakfast was never a meal of our ancestors. It was a notion made famous (and profitable) for the rich and wealthy class. A single full meal at a convenient time during the day is what our ancestors lived and thrived with. Intermittent fasting is just trying to bring back what was accepted as the perceived way of life by our ancestors.

Lunch

Now, let's look at the history of lunch. From the ancient Roman times until the Middle Ages, everyone ate around midday, and they called this primary meal dinner. The word or concept of 'lunch' did not exist. The day itself was structured very differently from what it is today. People rose earlier and went to bed earlier too than what we do today.

By midday, most workers during the Middle Ages would have already toiled for over 6 hours and would take a short break to eat a meal called 'luncheon' which was typically comprised of a big chunk of bread with a little cheese. Slowly, with the discovery of artificial light, dinner was pushed for later evening, especially for the richer class. Therefore, a light meal was needed during the day, and this was the precursor of what we know as lunch today.

The concept of 'lunch' was crystallized further during the Industrial Revolution when the working hours for the lower and middle class came to be clearly defined. Most of these people worked long hours in factories, and a noon-time meal became a necessity to sustain them efficiently throughout the day. Taking lunch slowly but surely became an ingrained daily habit for everybody in the western world.

Dinner

Dinner was a meal that existed even during the times of the ancient Romans, although the time of the meal was different from what we are normally accustomed to this day. The Romans called it the 'cena' which is Latin for dinner. While the aristocracy ate lavish, formal meals around noon time were attended to by many servants, and the meal cooked by many cooks, the peasantry ate around the same time although their food spreads were far more subdued and modest.

With natural light fading as the evening came, food was neither cooked nor eaten after sunset. With the advent and spread of artificial lighting, the time of dinner came to be pushed to the evenings. Moreover, the concept of lunch also started which pushed dinner to a later time of the day.

Towards the end of the 18th century, most people fit three meals into the day, especially where towns and cities were structured and long working hours became the norm. By the beginning of the 19th century, for most people dinner was a meal that was consumed after returning from a hectic day of work.

And, that is how three meals became a norm for everyone in the Western world. Now, it has been accepted as a way of eating for most of the communities around the globe. And aside from these three meals of breakfast, lunch, and dinner, a mid-morning snack and a mid-afternoon snack were added by a few people, taking the number of meals up to five a day!

The modern-day intermittent fasting is only formalizing

a habit that was followed by our ancestors until about three to four centuries ago. In addition to the convenience of having to worry about only 2-3 meals a day, the fact that there are multiple other benefits of intermittent fasting is proved by modern science. These benefits were already leveraged by our ancestors unwittingly or otherwise. Therefore, intermittent fasting is not a new phenomenon. It has always been the way our ancestors ate. They did it as a usual way of eating and we are simply giving it a new terminology, that's all.

Read on for a more detailed explanation on this ancient method of feeding our body.

Chapter 1

History of Fasting

The history of fasting cannot really have a clear starting point because there is no reason to believe that early man did not fast in a natural way. Not just humans, even animals abstain from eating when they fall ill or are physically discomforted in any way. It is a natural reaction of all living organisms to rest and conserve energy during times of illness.

Fasting and Ancient Greeks

The ancient wise men of Greece took lessons from nature to find cures for human sickness. Fasting is an inherent instinct that prevents all living beings, including humans and animals, to become anorexic when they feel ill. It is easy to believe this because all you need is to think back to the last time you had the flu. Eating would have been the last thing on your mind. In fact, the thought of food creates a nauseous feeling when you are sick. Therefore, fasting is a universal instinct of life to protect itself during an illness. It would be quite right to say that fasting is ingrained in the human psyche and is as old as mankind.

Even before the advent of modern medicine, fasting was considered a natural healing mechanism. Hippocrates, the ancient Greek doctor, and philosopher who is regarded as the father of modern medicine not only prescribed but also championed the practice of fasting. He advised consuming apple cider vinegar during the fasting period. One of his famous quotes about fasting is, "When you eat during an illness, you are, in effect, feeding your illness."

Another ancient Greek philosopher and writer, Plutarch, also believed in the efficacy of fasting to treat sickness. He wrote, 'It would be better if you fasted instead of taking any medicines today." Other Greek philosophers and staunch followers and supporters of fasting were Plato, and his famous student, Aristotle.

Moreover, the ancient philosophers of Greece also believed that fasting improves thinking and cognitive abilities. This again would have been experienced by many of us. Can you recall how you felt after a huge meal during a festival such as Christmas or Thanksgiving? After consuming that big meal, did you feel highly energetic or lethargic to the point of wanting to simply lie down? It is quite likely the latter answer.

When you overeat, a lot more blood is pumped into the digestive system to help it manage the large influx of food resulting in a lesser amount of blood reaching your brain. The result is referred to as a 'food coma.'

Herbert Shelton (1895 – 1985), the world-renowned naturopath, an advocate of alternative medicine, and a vegetarian, oversaw fasting and cleansing treatments of over 40,000 patients during his lifetime. He said, "Fasting should be recognized as the oldest form of treating and caring for sick organisms based on the plane of instinct." It is easy to believe this physician because you only need to look back in your life to notice how many times you have abstained from eating when you are sick because you just could not bear to consume any food. You did not need a qualified doctor to understand your instinct to abstain from food during an illness.

Dr. Shelton has written over 40 books on various aspects of health, and one of his bestsellers is *The Science and Fine Art of Fasting*. As early as the 1940s, he advocated a treatment where water fasting was a primary mode of therapy.

Paracelsus, a Renaissance period doctor, considered to be one of the three founders (the other two being Hippocrates and Galen) of modern medicine is believed to have said that fasting is the best remedy for many illnesses. He called fasting as the 'physician within.' Early healing practices recognized and respected the revitalizing power of fasting.

Benjamin Franklin, another intellectual giant of the 18th century who had mastered many subjects, wrote, 'Fasting and resting are the best of all medicines."

Religion and Fasting

Early spiritual and religious groups employed fasting as a means of purification before conducting any rites and ceremonies. In many of the tribal cultures, fasting was often a necessary element for soldiers to indulge in before setting off for a battle. Many North American tribes used fasting as a form of prayer seeking divine protection against natural catastrophes such as famines and floods. From time immemorial, fasting has always been connected to an attitude of self-control, sacrifice, and penitence.

Catholicism

In contemporary times, fasting in Catholicism is usually taken in the form of one large meal, and one or two smaller meals, all of which will add up to less than the non-fasting days' meals. Ideally, no food should be consumed between the meals fixed for fasting days. This kind of fast is typically enforced during the time of Lent, the penitential 40-day period before Easter. Some Catholics fast every Friday or Wednesdays and Saturdays. There is also the Ember Days kept aside for fasting and prayers that some of the Catholics around the world follow.

All these fasting practices mentioned have been toned down and become significantly less strict over time. The 'Black Fast' was one of the most rigorous fasts of Catholicism followed during the Lent period. The 'Black Fast' consisted of only one meal a day to be consumed after sunset.

Even this one meal of the day was very restricted regarding what could be eaten and what could not. Meat, alcohol, eggs, and dairy were strictly prohibited. Additionally, during the Holy Week, the meal consisted only of bread and water with some herbs and salt.

Over time, especially in the Western world, the strictness of the fast reduced significantly. During the 14th century, the post-sunset meal was moved to lunch time to which was added an evening snack. By the 19th century, a morning snack was also allowed, and in the 20th century, it was even allowed to replace fasting with charity and prayers.

Catholics on the eastern side of the globe follow stricter norms of fasting, restricting their food consumption to one meal a day, and abstaining from animal products.

Mormonism

Mormons have a concept of community fasting and prayer day, usually on the first Sunday of each month, referred to as 'fasting Sunday.' It is usually a collective exercise in which all families including children above the age of eight years are encouraged to fast. The 'fasting Sunday' entails skipping two consecutive meals in a 24-hour period. The money that is believed to have been saved by skipping the two meals is typically donated to charity, called the 'fast offering.'

Islam

The Five Pillars of Islam include a declaration of faith, charity, prayer, pilgrimage, and fasting. Ramadan is observed for an entire month each year. During the month of Ramadan, no food is allowed to be consumed during daylight. Smoking and alcohol are also strictly forbidden. Other than the obligatory Ramadan fasting period, there are multiple non-obligatory days such as all Mondays and Thursdays on which fasting can be observed. Fasting is forbidden on certain holy days when feasting is involved.

In the Islam religion, fasting is typically started with an intention, which can be a private matter for each person or family. If for some reason, the fast is broken on a day, one must fast on an additional day. In the olden times of slavery, if the fast is broken with sex, then the penalties were stricter. The person must free a slave or clothe/feed 60 people or fast for another two months.

In Islam, fasting is believed to bring people closer to God

while creating a sense of comradeship and solidarity with fellow fasting members of the community. It helps you empathize with the less fortunate people of the world, and also acts as an exercise to build self-control. However, Islam believes that mere fasting in the absence of any spiritual intention is nothing more than starvation.

Judaism

The traditional Jews fast on six days spread across the year. On these fasting days, no food or drink is allowed from sunset of one day to the sunset of the following day (a 24-hour fasting window). Two of these six days is Tisha B'Av and Yom Kippur. On these two days, in addition to fasting, other restrictions including wearing leather, washing and cleaning your body, sexual interaction, and using perfume also apply. The other four of the six days do not have these restrictions.

Buddhism

Monks who are called bhikkhus and bhikkhunis follow the Vinyana rule which forbids them to eat anything after the noon meal. This means the Buddhist monks' daily regimen consists of only one meal at noon time. The monks do not treat this as fasting. They only consider it their daily routine that helps in maintaining good health and aids meditation.

The lay Buddhist chooses to follow this fast on six days of each month. The purpose of this fast for the common individual who follows Buddhism is to demonstrate compassion for the ones who are starving by 'reducing their share of food.' For Buddhists, fasting is also a form of moderation, a concept practiced and preached by Lord Buddha. So, eating less on six days of the month helps them achieve moderation in their food consumption.

Primarily, the concept of fasting in Buddhism is to cleanse the human body and to bring in clarity in thought. Fasting in Buddhism includes mostly having one full meal by noon after which liquids are permitted. Eating at night is typically not allowed on fasting days.

Hinduism

Vratas are a form of religious obligation that Hindus follow. One such vrata consists of partial or complete fasting during which time in addition to abstaining from or restricting intake of food, the practitioners must remain pure in body and mind, do not utter lies, practice tolerance and control of their anger, and perform certain rites and rituals.

On two particular days of the lunar month (referred to as Ekadashi), Hindus fast for 36 hours starting from the sunset of the previous day of Ekadashi up to the sunrise after the day of Ekadashi. During this time, typically, the only food consumed is in the form of whole fruits or fruit juices. All these types of fasts have reduced in strictness and intensity over time.

Jainism

The followers of Jainism are called Jains and fasting is a common religious aspect in their lives. A regular fasting mechanism that is almost a daily routine in Jainism is not to eat until satiation. Full fasts in this religion involve complete abstinence from food and even water. Sometimes, the Jains consume boiled water during the fasting period. All Jains are also strict vegetarians.

Jainism advocates fasting primarily to keep bodily desires and needs in check thereby resolving bad karma and uplifting the soul. During the period of fasting, the Jains are expected to pray, serve the nuns and monks, meditate, read scriptures, and perform charitable deeds. Fasting in Jainism is typically performed on the 8th and the 14th days of the lunar cycle and for a week before the advent of any festival.

It is evident that nearly all religions of the world employ the idea of fasting in some form or the other. The reasons for fasting are many including but not limited to:

- To get closer to God.

- To empathize with the less fortunate people who

go hungry more often than they should.

- As a form of penance, sacrifice, or mourning.

- To achieve spiritual enlightenment.

- To simply break the unhealthy habit of gluttony.

- To help in the physical and spiritual healing process.

Whatever is the reason, fasting triggers self-reflection in us driving us to see things more deeply than if we were completely stuffed or satiated. If the concept of religion is taken away from the act of fasting, self-denial in a conscious way gives us a sense of achievement at the end of the exercise. Fasting helps us understand our level of self-control and willpower, and how we can work on improving these two essential character-building personality traits.

A Brief Glimpse on Modern Day Fasting

In the modern day, many physicians do recommend fasting as a way of healing your body. While conventional modern medicine is still working on various studies to prove/disprove the efficacies of fasting, many healthcare professionals are optimistic about intermittent fasting.

Moreover, as more studies prove the deep connection that exists between the body and mind, modern-day physicians are opening up to the concept of fasting within reasonable limits. These conventional doctors are becoming attuned to the idea of an 'internal' influence within our mind which is committed to incline our body and mind towards health and balance.

These doctors are open to the idea (based on multiple body-mind scientific experiments) that we can harness this 'internal' influence to correct and heal our systems in a natural way with lesser effects of harmful chemicals. These set of doctors are continuously working across the globe to prove that the body is not just a set of biological processes but goes beyond the physical aspect that we feel and easily experience.

Interestingly, most doctors agree that the best of medicine and surgery cannot cure or treat someone who is not emotionally, physically, and spiritually inclined towards healing. A large part of effective healing is based on the person's desire to be healed. All scientists agree that only the human body has the power to restore injured tissues to their original state of perfection. External medicines contribute significantly to repairing damaged physical parts of the body but can never achieve the original perfection on their own. They need the emotional and spiritual help from the body and mind of the afflicted person.

Medications only facilitate the process to take place

faster and with less pain. In fact, many physicians agree on the fact that the natural healing remedies of our ancestors effectively geared our spiritual and emotional aspects towards health. Fasting is the perfect example of such natural remedies. A simple 1-day fast can potentially change the way your body and mind respond to hunger pangs.

Even today, the Fasting Institutes set up by Dr. Herbert Shelton are very popular and people frequently visit for various fasting-based treatments.

Fasting Vs Starvation

One of the biggest misconceptions about fasting is that it is considered the same as starvation. Although they seem to be similar, there are distinct differences between the two. Let's discuss the differences to prevent any confusion between fasting and starvation.

The Basics of Fasting – Fasting entails abstinence from food and drinks (except water, perhaps) for a specific and limited period of time. Fasting is recommended for many medical cases including testing for blood sugar levels, before and after surgeries, and other similar instances. Fasting involves planning and it is completely voluntary and controlled. Intake of nutrients may be withheld for some time to achieve the desired result. But, there is never a complete absence of essential nutrients in your body.

The Basics of Starvation – Starvation, on the other hand, is a severe, or even total, lack of essential nutrients needed for the sustenance of human life. Starvation can be a result of a lack of important nutrients such as proteins, carbs, fats, and other vital elements or can also be a result of not consuming sufficient liquids. Starvation is involuntary and irrational and could be based on the non-availability of food and drinks. There is no benefits of starvation.

A classic analogy to illustrate the difference between starvation and fasting is dying of old age and committing suicide. Starvation is akin to committing suicide whereas fasting is dying of old age after living a healthy and happy life.

Fasting or abstention from food deliberately and voluntarily under the supervision of a trained medical professional is the art of manipulating the metabolic system to achieve specific desired outcomes. However, fasting in a malpractice scenario can seem like starvation. Fasting correctly and in an effective way can do a lot of good to the body and mind.

During the fasting mode, our body systematically cleanses itself of nearly everything except the vital tissues. The body continuously readjusts itself to make very little demand on the stored reserves. Starvation occurs only when the body begins to utilize its vital tissues for sustenance. Human beings, like other living organisms, can adapt extremely well to the lack of food.

In extreme cases (which is only used as an illustration and not for trying at home without supervision), there are cases of people surviving for up to 75 days on water fasting! Here is a quick analysis of how this is possible. Every pound of human fat is worth approximately 3500 calories. Each extra pound of fat that we carry around can effectively supply our body enough calories to last us an entire day filled with intense physical labor!

While being able to use all the excess fat in our body only through fasting calls for immense (almost demonic) willpower and mental strength to manage and overcome the myriad body symptoms, it is possible. Again, this kind of extreme fasting should never be done at home without medical supervision. But, there are many strictly-supervised cases where people have been able to fast and lose their excess fat effectively.

The most important difference between fasting and starvation is the severity of symptoms one experiences when abstaining from food and drinks. Fasting for a short while might initially cause temporary discomforts such as hunger pangs, headaches, lightheadedness, dizziness, and fatigue. People in starvation experience more severe symptoms such as heart convulsions, heart failure, brain dysfunction, and more; all or any of which if not reversed can quickly become fatal. The longer the period of fasting, the closer the symptoms will be to that of starvation.

The concept of fasting appears difficult to sustain and seemingly unscientific in the modern times, especially in the western world, because calorie-rich food is available in plenty, and relatively easily. It is so much easier to reach out to food when the first pangs of hunger hit you instead of using your willpower to stop yourself from eating when your body does not necessarily need any food. This situation results in a scenario wherein unless there is a famine or you are involved in a strenuous exercise regimen on a daily basis, it is almost impossible to burn up the entire accumulated fat content in our body.

Breakfast is an example of a meal that breaks the fast that your body was unwittingly undergoing while you were asleep. The nightly fasting regimen of your body is a natural cleansing miracle that our system has developed. When you wake up from this short fast, you will notice you have foul breath, your tongue is coated with something unpleasant, your skin is puffy, and your mind is foggy. Well, these are all nothing but early and temporary symptoms of fasting during which time your body has been in a state of detoxification. A good breakfast will remove all these symptoms, and you think you have done yourself a great job.

After you read this book, you will see how great it is for you to extend this fasting period for a little longer and allow your body to complete its detoxification process before feeding yourself. Intermittent fasting, because that is what extending the time of breaking your night fast is all about, will not need much medical supervision because you are going to replenish your body with required nutrients soon afterwards. Read on to find out more about intermittent fasting.

A word of caution at this point is in order. It would be a wise decision to seek professional help or at least talk to your physician before you jump into fasting. Ideally, fasts that are restricted to five days or less are safe to be done at home though if you are taking medications of any kind whatsoever, medical supervision is strictly recommended.

Chapter 2

Intermittent Fasting

We learned in the previous chapter how fasting is as old as mankind or even life itself. It is used by all animals and human beings to rest and recuperate their body systems.

What Is Intermittent Fasting?

Before the standard 3-4 meals came into play for human beings, our ancestors (say about 2000-3000 years ago) did nothing but switch between fasting and feasting. They did not have easy access to food, and during these difficult days, they simply fasted. Then, someone in the group would kill a large animal, and they had to eat the meat quickly before it started to rot. During these happy days, our ancestors feasted.

Intermittent fasting is nothing but fasting and feasting alternately with the periods varying in length. The primary focus of intermittent fasting is not on what you eat but when you eat although what you eat is also an important factor for successful results when fasting. You don't have to worry too much about nutrients such as micromanaging how much carbs, proteins, fats, etc.

should be in your meal. Also, there is not much focus on what foods to avoid except excessive junk and unprocessed foods. Intermittent fasting is not a diet but is only a method or pattern of eating.

You only control the time when you choose to eat your meals. Intermittent fasting (IF) is an eating schedule that alternates between feeding and fasting. You set two windows; one for eating and one for fasting. We will start the explanation with breakfast. Breakfast is an almost glorified meal of the day in these modern times.

Various cereal-manufacturing companies urge you to eat a 'healthy wholesome' breakfast to keep your energy levels high throughout the day. In retrospect, this concept of not skipping breakfast seems to be more of an effective marketing campaign than teaching consumers how to eat healthily. Many studies reveal that skipping breakfast might actually be a good thing.

Intermittent fasting tells you to skip breakfast because it allows your body to remain in the fasted state for a longer period of time. Remaining in the fasted state is where all of the benefits of intermittent fasting reside. A classic example of a daily intermittent fasting method is to have an eating window between 12 noon and 8 pm. After your 8 pm meal, you fast until the next day at 12 noon.

One of the primary reasons for the increasing popularity of intermittent fasting is because it is quite easy to stick to. It does not restrict you from eating any of your favorite foods. Of course, an important caveat is to maintain calorie deficiency if you are using this method to lose weight and extra waist inches.

Intermittent fasting works differently for different people; like any other form of dieting or eating pattern. Some people find it difficult, at least initially, to get into the rhythm while for some others, fitting the intermittent fasting schedule into their lifestyle is not just easy but makes their life more convenient too. Fortunately, this pattern of eating is so flexible that it offers novices to start and advance at their own pace.

It is perfectly fine if you choose to ease yourself into it over a long duration during which time the concept of intermittent fasting would have become a deeply ingrained habit for you. Alternately, if it suits you, you can jump straight in and start off on a daily 16:8 pattern and increase the intensity depending on your ability to manage hunger pangs.

Basics of Human Metabolism

Before we get into the deep end of intermittent fasting, and how it works, let us understand the basics of the human metabolism. Our food is essentially composed of three macronutrients including carbohydrates, proteins, and fats. Different foods have different percentages of these macronutrients in them.

For example, sugar, honey, rice, pasta, bread, etc. have a high content of carbohydrates whereas fish, meat, and eggs are mostly proteins. Similarly, cooking oils, butter, ghee, etc. are rich in fats. Some foods such as cakes, fried foods, and biscuits also have a high content of fats and carbohydrates.

The process of metabolism starts after we have consumed food, and the starting point of metabolism is the breaking down of these macronutrients into their component elements. These macronutrients are broken down into the following energy forms:

- Carbohydrates are broken down into glucose or simple sugars.

- Proteins' basic elements are amino acids.

- Fats get converted to fatty acids.

Glucose and fatty acids are then used by our body as the primary source of fuel and energy while amino acids are essentially used for repair and maintenance. All the excess energy forms are stored for later use. How do these three nutrient components (glucose, fatty acids, and amino acids) work in our body? Let's take a closer look.

Glucose – Typically, after a meal, the blood glucose level rises rapidly which, in turn, triggers the production and release of an important digestive hormone called insulin. The primary responsibility of insulin is to transport blood glucose to other body parts and tissues for use as energy fuel.

All the surplus glucose which is not immediately needed by your body get converted into glycogen and stored in liver and muscles. The space in your muscles and liver is very limited, and so, the rest of the surplus glucose gets converted into fats and is stored as fat reserves (or adipose tissues) all over the body.

Amino Acids – are essentially used by the body for repair and maintenance. Most adults need very little amino acids for repair purposes, and any surplus also gets accumulated in the liver as glycogen.

Fatty Acids – Unless you have not consumed carbohydrates at all, the fats are typically not needed by your body for immediate use. A very small amount of fatty acids are needed along with amino acids for repair and maintenance work. So, the rest (which is nearly all) are fats you have consumed in your meal and get stored as adipose tissues all over the body.

Therefore, after eating, our body is busy storing away excess nutrients in the form of fat or adipose tissues. This entire process lasts several hours after each meal. Considering the frequency of our meals, the metabolic process of one meal invariably overlaps into that of the next meal, and so forth.

The only time this process comes to a complete halt in your body is when you have not eaten for a long time, and your body turned to the 'fasted state.' During the fasted state, your body does not store any excess fat but uses the stored fat for its fuel. That is the basis of losing fat with intermittent fasting.

How Does Intermittent Fasting Work?

Our body can be only in two states; fasted and fed (or feasting). Let's look at each of these states in a bit of detail to understand the working of intermittent fasting better.

Fed or Feasting State – After you have eaten a meal, it remains in your body for a couple of hours, and it takes any time between 8-12 hours for the nutrients from the consumed food to be completely processed. During these 8-12 hours, your body breaks down the consumed food into its constituent nutrients which are then absorbed.

During the feasting state, the primary source of energy for your body is from this consumed food. Therefore, your body uses up the energy provided by the food eaten in your last meal for all of its activities and will not use any of the stored energy during this period.

Fasted State – After about 8-12 hours from your last meal, your body gets into a fasted state. This 8-12 fasting state is normal for most of us because we don't eat anything when we are sleeping at night. But, as soon as we get up, invariably we have our breakfast.

For hundreds and thousands of years before the concept of breakfast came into our lives, working normally in a fasted state was an accepted thing for humans. It still is for animals because you don't find them eating breakfast as soon as they get up. During this fasted state, our bodies burn up the stored fat for use as energy fuel.

Intermittent fasting is nothing but a deliberate and conscious effort to keep our bodies in the fasted state for longer and more frequent periods than just skipping breakfast. In addition to the burning up of stored fat for energy, there are multiple other benefits intermittent fasting offers all of which are discussed in Chapter 4.

Myths Surrounding Intermittent Fasting

Like most popular elements of the world, intermittent fasting too has its share of myths that need to be broken to clearly and unambiguously understand the way it operates. So, let's go and bust some myths.

Intermittent fasting will lead us into

starvation mode –People are led to believe that intermittent fasting will put our bodies into a starvation mode because our brain gets the signal that it is 'famine time' lowering its rate of metabolism. This is nothing but a myth. Studies have shown that our bodies do not lower their metabolic rates unless and until you have not given it nourishment for at least three entire days.

Since our cavemen days, the human body has been developed to withstand days of famine. How can a few hours of not eating anything put your body on the defensive? I would like to reiterate a subsection of Chapter 1 under Starvation Vs Fasting. Starvation mode starts only when the body has completely used up all its fat reserves. Only at this stage will our body break down muscle. Muscles will not be touched by your body if you skipped a meal or two, and definitely not if you have only skipped breakfast!

Intermittent fasting compels your body to use up stored fat while keeping your lean mass intact. If you have excessive fat in your body, then intermittent fasting can work wonders because it will reach out for these reserves almost immediately after it has completely utilized the energy from your last meal.

Intermittent fasting gives you the freedom to eat whatever you want during the eating

window – Unfortunately, this myth is also the biggest pitfall for novices to fall into as they struggle to make intermittent fasting work. Yes, you have fasted for a certain period. But, that does not give you the freedom to eat whatever you want once the fasting period is over.

Losing weight from intermittent fasting is also based on a caloric deficit. If you exceed your daily calorie needs, you will never lose weight. The number of calories that your body continuously burns throughout the day to maintain your current body weight is what is referred to as daily calorific needs.

Your daily calorie intake is dependent on a whole lot of factors including your age, gender, body fat, weight, height, physical activity levels, profession, and more. If you consume more calories than what your body burns during your eating window, then you will gain weight irrespective of how long you fasted for before it.

You must be watchful of how many calories you are consuming to ensure you stay within the required range. Additionally, your meals must include plenty of fresh fruits and vegetables to meet your body's fiber needs. Excessively fatty foods, processed foods, food with preservatives should be avoided. Nutritious, wholesome, and fresh foods are your best bet.

Intermittent fasting will make you feel hungry always – A great worry that people have about intermittent fasting is that they will have to stay hungry for 16, 18 or even 20 hours. In the minds of novices, this means being hungry almost every minute of the day! This is a total myth.

Initially, intermitting fasting is going to make you uncomfortable because your body has got accustomed to receiving food at frequent intervals, and hasn't got an opportunity to reach out to the stored fat reserves. Your body and mind are going to take a little bit of time in getting used to the paradigm shift in energy consumption.

But, once your body understands that the energy reserves are right there for it to take (and, plenty of it, too), it will cease to create unpleasant and uncomfortable sensations for you. Your body will automatically shift its metabolic mechanism to adapt to your new eating methods. Hunger pangs will disappear after the initial adjustment.

Starting slowly is a great way to manage hunger pangs. Start with the 12-hour fasting period, then move to the 14-hour period, and then to the 16-hour period. This way, your body will not unduly send out hunger pangs signals. Always listen to what your body is telling you and move forward gradually for maximum effect. The 18-hour period should typically be your ultimate aim. However, the 16:8 method can do wonders too.

Intermittent fasting is a 'magical' trick –

Nothing can be farther from the truth. Yes, it might seem like magic considering the quick and effective results it can produce. But, multiple scientific studies have proven the efficacy of intermittent fasting in bringing about the desired outcomes using basic human metabolism.

Moreover, you already know that fasting is not some new-age weight-loss dieting cult. It has been around for thousands of years as a natural healing and cleansing process. The recent scientific studies only support what our ancestors already knew and followed on a day-to-day basis.

The basic science behind intermittent fasting is simple. If you spend more calories than you consume, your body will be in caloric deficit. And, it will use up fat reserves for the differential energy resulting in fat/weight loss. If the value of one pound of fat is 3500 calories, then reducing 500 calories from your base metabolic rate will result in a loss of one pound of weight every week.

The science behind intermittent fasting is discussed in detail in the next section of this chapter.

Intermittent fasting is just another crash/fad diet – One of the first things you learned about intermittent fasting is that it is not a diet. It is only a pattern of eating. Theoretically, as long as you consume fewer calories than what you spend, your meal can be pizza and beer too. However, in practice, this approach will not work because eating only pizza and beer will never help you get all the essential nutrients your body needs for healthy living.

Intermittent fasting is, therefore, only a guide and tells you clearly WHEN you should NOT eat. It is not a fad or crash diet that promises you miracles if you stay away from or eat certain types of food.

The Science Behind Intermittent Fasting

Glucose and fat are the two primary sources of energy for our body. Since glucose is more easily broken down than fat, our body, by default, chooses glucose over fat when both are available. But, if glucose is not available, the body can easily turn to fat for its energy needs, and that too, without any harmful effect.

At the very basic level, intermittent fasting compels your body to burn off the excess fat into energy to meet its calorie requirements in the absence of food. What is body fat? It is nothing but excess energy from food that is stored away. If you don't consume, your body will simply 'eat' the stored fat for its energy needs.

Insulin is one of the most critical hormones associated with food digestion. The level of insulin in your bloodstream increases when you eat. Insulin facilitates the storage of food energy in two ways. First, simple sugars are converted into glycogen and stored in the liver. The liver may be resembled to your refrigerator in which it is easy to store and access food; but, there is limited space.

Second, owing to limited storage space in the liver,

glycogen gets converted into fat which is then taken to other parts of the body and stored as fat deposits. The transfer and deposition of fat is a complex process. But, there is no limit on the amount of fat that your body can store.

Your body can be compared to a large freezer in which storing food is difficult to store and access. The food stored in that freezer will remain, and if not removed or taken care of, can turn toxic, just like your fat deposits. The trick in any health-focused regimen whether it is a diet or fast is to work on and access the freezer.

Therefore, there are two alternate sources of energy in our body. One is in the form of glycogen (limited amount) in the liver, and the second one is in the form of fat deposits all over the body. The glycogen is easily accessible whereas the fat is more difficult to access as it is spread all over the body.

Now, when the body is in a fasting state, the level of insulin in the blood gets reduced. This reduction in insulin will signal the body to start burning stored energy to meet its energy requirements the body does not receive food. The glucose level in the blood falls which means the body will draw stored glycogen from the liver. When this stored glycogen supply is consumed, the body will turn to stored fat for its energy needs.

Our body, therefore, exists in only two states; the fed state where insulin levels are high and the fasting state where insulin levels are low. In the fed state, our body is storing food energy and in the fasting state, our body is burning this energy. It's always one state or the other. If we balance the fed and fasting states, there will be no weight gain.

Look at the typical modern-day scenario. We start eating from the minute we get up from sleep in the morning and continue to feed ourselves until we go back to sleep at night. This fed state is continuously storing food energy. There is very little fasting time given to the body to use up this stored energy. Your body will never get an opportunity to burn up the stored energy because you are constantly supplying it with food.

There is no balance between the fed and the fasting state resulting in weight gain. Intermittent fasting helps you regain the essential balance between the fed and the fasting states thereby helping you lead a healthier life than before.

During fasting states, it is not only fats that are being broken. Realistically, our body uses a combination of fats (from adipose tissues), ketones (from the fatty acids of the liver), and glucose made from glycogen (in liver and muscles) for its energy during the fasting state. All these forms of energy are needed because different tissues require different kinds of fuel:

- The muscles use the glucose from the glycogen stored in them for energy or fats from adipose tissues.

- The heart functions excellently with fats.

- Nerves and the brain prefer work most efficiently with glucose though they can use ketones too.

- Red blood cells need only glucose and ketones or fatty acids cannot be used by them.

Therefore, the body needs to maintain sufficient blood-sugar levels for the RBCs to do their work and for the brain to function properly. During fasting, this glucose has been converted and stored from the liver into sugar through a process called glycogenolysis. The liver is also capable of converting stored fat and amino acids into glucose.

The process of metabolism in our body is quite complex, and it is important to remember that it needs all three macronutrients to function efficiently. Fasting empowers our metabolic system to leverage the power of stored fat for nearly all its energy purposes.

Hormonal Changes due to Intermittent Fasting

Fasting triggers many changes at the hormonal level in our body. Let's look at some of the important hormones that get affected by fasting.

Insulin – is an essential hormone that comes into active play after a meal. Insulin's primary task is to use up glucose from our food as energy or get it stored away as fat. Glucose should not remain in the bloodstream for a long time. Keeping the blood-sugar level in our body in a healthy range is essential because the accumulation of glucose is toxic and can damage our body.

If insulin does not function properly, then the high levels of glucose in the bloodstream can damage many tissues in our body including nerves, blood vessels, eyes, kidneys, etc. This is the beginning of diabetes. The job of insulin is to convert glucose to fat for storage purposes, and therefore, when there is a lot of insulin in the blood, fat reserves can never be used as body fuel.

Fasting is, perhaps, the oldest and the most effective way to reduce the level of insulin in our body. Intake of food raises insulin levels and, therefore, reducing intake or fasting is the best way to decrease insulin levels. Interestingly, when the body switches over to fat metabolism in the absence of glucose, the blood glucose level remains normal during short-term fasting; less than

36 hours.

In addition to directly reducing the insulin levels in the blood, fasting also facilitates increased sensitivity to insulin thereby reducing the need for greater levels of this weight-gaining hormone. When insulin is reduced, excess water and salt are also drained out from the body resulting in more weight loss.

Glucagon – This hormone's job is to bring back the level of glucose if it has dropped very low. Also, glucagon ensures that there is sufficient supply of energy for our body. During fasting, it achieves this purpose by stimulating the release of stored glycogen into glucose, manufacture glucose from fat reserves and from stored amino acids, and to release fat from fat reserves. Therefore, during fasting, the body is compelled by various sources to burn fat.

Growth Hormones – facilitate increased usage of fat for energy while preserving bone density and muscle mass. The secretion of this critical hormone reduces with age. Fasting is proven to be one of the best stimuli that improve the secretion of growth hormones. Growth hormones are also an essential element for the cell renewal process.

Electrolytes – One of the major concerns about fasting is the loss of micronutrients. However, studies have proven that even prolonged fasting (up to 2 months) does not affect the stability of critical electrolytes such as potassium, calcium, magnesium, and phosphorus in our body. The reason attributed to this stable level is that most of the electrolytes are stored in the bones which are not affected by intermittent fasting in any way.

Noradrenaline – levels are increased which is one of the important reasons for improved energy levels during intermittent fasting. Many studies reveal that contrary to the misplaced fear of metabolic shut-down during fasting, a 48-hour fasting increases metabolic rate by 3.6%.

Interestingly, fasting produces many hormonal changes that are beneficial to us. Essentially, fasting compels the body to turn to fat instead of glucose for its fuel needs. We are effectively 'eating' our own fat during fasting which can only be good for us. Our metabolic rate is increased during fasting.

The fasting process compels your body to reach out to the ample energy source accumulated in the 'freezer,' or fat, instead of choosing the easier option of accessing consumed food from the 'refrigerator,' or glucose

Intermittent fasting is, therefore, an effective, ancient way of managing our metabolism naturally by inhibiting intake of calories instead of trying to give alternate, and seemingly healthy, sources of calories. Intermittent fasting is a straightforward approach to weight loss and a healthy life; it is like taking the bull by its horns.

Chapter 3

Types and Basic Pros and Cons of Intermittent Fasting

There are various types of intermittent fasting which is one of the reasons for its flexibility of use. Depending on your suitability, you can choose one or more methods. You could start with the easiest and most popular method, and slowly advance to more difficult options at your pace.

Types of Intermittent Fasting

The 12-12 Method

This is the easiest and the most popular method of intermittent fasting and is perfect for beginners. You could already be in this schedule unwittingly. In this method, you have an eating window of 12 hours and a fasting window of 12 hours.

So, if your dinner time is 8 pm and you have breakfast the next morning at 8 am, then you are already on this schedule, and you don't even know it. If you have been snacking after dinner, you should stop it immediately. For beginners, this method is great to get your body and mind strict about eating and feasting windows.

The 16:8 Method

This is also achievable by most novices. However, it can be a huge challenge for people who don't like to miss dinner AND breakfast. The keyword here is 'AND.' For this method to be a success, you must be ready to skip one of these two meals. By skipping one of the two meals, you will get a 16-hour fasting window which includes your 8-hour sleeping time. Your feeding window will be a balance of 8 hours a day.

For people who have never fasted before, this method could be a great starting point. Finish your dinner by 8 pm and get to bed by 10 pm. When you wake up at 6 am the next morning, 10 hours of the fasting period is already done. Skip breakfast, and you can have your first meal of the day at 12 noon. Just make sure you hydrate yourself well during the fasting window. Also you can drink tea or coffee, black and sugarless which can help fight hunger pangs.

Although initially, it might be tough, it does get easier as you persist. During the feasting window, you can fit in 2 or 3 meals. This method is referred to as the Leangains protocol and was made popular by Martin Berkhan, a famous fitness expert.

The dinner-skipping way of following the Leangains method involves an eating window from 8 am – 4 pm (your last meal of the day) and a fasting window of 4 pm – 8 am the next day. If 4 pm for your last meal is very far away from your bedtime, you can shift your eating to 10 am (your first meal of the day) to 6 pm (your last meal of the day). Here is a small chart to help you understand how you can plan your 16:8 daily intermittent fasting schedules:

- If your first meal is at 7AM, your last meal should be at 3pm.

- If your first meal is at 8AM, your last meal should be at 4pm.

- If your first meal is at 11AM, your last meal should be at 7pm.

- If your first meal is at 2PM, your last meal should be at 10pm.

The 18:6 Method

This method will test your willpower a little more than

the 16:8 method. It is definitely more difficult to achieve than the previous method as you need to gather all your mental strength and fight off hunger pangs for 18 hours; 2 hours more than 16! Moreover, with an eating window of only 6 hours, you cannot get more than 2 meals, and perhaps, squeeze in one little snack in-between.

The good thing about this method is once you have perfected it and your body and mind have come to accept it as part of your life, you don't have to try any more extreme intermittent fasting methods. The 18:6 method will suffice for the rest of your life.

You can extend each day's fasting regimen to cover more hours for fasting and lesser hours for eating. For example, you could have a fasting window for 20 hours and an eating window of 4 hours (20:4, tough yes, but doable over a long period of time). Or, you could have one meal a day in which you ensure you get all the nutrients your body needs.

The last two methods are really extreme and cannot be done on a daily basis. You can keep them for special days to test your mental strength and willpower capacity. Even the keenest fasting advocates might not be able to manage the 20:4 and one-meal-a-day on a consistent basis.

Additionally, any extreme fasting method to be maintained for more than a couple of days should never be attempted without medical supervision.

The 5:2 Diet

This method of intermittent fasting entails following a normal eating pattern (without any fasting schedule) on 5 days of the week and restricting calorie intake to 500-600 calories on two days. This diet is called the Fast Diet and was made popular by Michael Mosley, a British doctor and journalist. Women are advised to consume 500 calories and men 600 calories on the two fasting days of the week.

A great example of the 5:2 diet would be to restrict calorie intake on Mondays and Thursdays, and eating normally on all the other days. You can choose any two days that are suitable for you. However, the most effective way of doing this fast is to choose two consecutive fasting days when you will restrict your calorie intake to 500-600. Your metabolism will highly benefit by this method of fasting, especially if you can manage two consecutive fasting days instead of two separate days.

The 24-Hour Fast

While eating one meal a day on a regular basis is not just difficult but also not highly advised, fasting one day a week for 24 hours is doable and a great intermittent fasting method too. Brad Pilon, another famous fitness expert, advocated and popularized this method of intermittent fasting.

Dinner at 7 pm on Monday followed by dinner at 7 pm on Tuesday is an example of the 24-hour fasting method. You could also choose to do breakfast-to-breakfast or lunch-to-lunch. During the 24-hour fasting period, only tea, coffee, and other non-calorie liquids are allowed.

The trick to making a success of this intermittent fasting method is to stick to eating normally on your first meal after the 24 hour fasting period. You must consume the same amount of food that you would have eaten had you not fasted. Again, staying in the fasting mode for 24 hours can be a huge challenge for many. The first few hours might go off uneventfully but later on, ravenous hunger can create a lot of temporary discomfort. You will have to give your best self-discipline ways to make this method a success.

However, you don't need to start off in such a rigorous way. Instead of starting off at the 24-hour level, you can start off at a 14-16 hour level on one day of the first week, and slowly increase it to 24 hours after 3-4 weeks or at your pace.

The Alternate-Day Fasting Method

This method requires you to fast every other day and eat normally every other day. On the fasting days, your calorie intake should be restricted to 500-600. The alternate-day fasting method calls for going hungry to bed several days each week which may not be an easy or pleasant thing to do and can be quite an extreme method.

The Warrior Diet

This method of intermittent fasting entails consuming:

- Fruits and raw vegetables in small quantities during the day.

- One big meal at dinner time.

Primarily, the warrior diet consists of fasting all day and feasting at one meal. However, it is different from the rigorous 24-hour fasting diet because here, you do consume fruits and vegetables which can be great to stave off hunger pangs effectively and in a healthy manner. The nighttime meal is typically similar to the paleo diet consisting of wholesome and unprocessed foods that are as close to how nature provides them as possible.

Despite the fruits and vegetables, the Warrior Diet can be quite a challenge and as beginners, it might not make sense to try it until you have understood how your body responds to easier methods of intermittent fasting.

Spontaneous Intermitting Fasting

This method does not have any structure or planning to it. You simply choose to skip one or two meals if you are not feeling hungry or do not have the time to cook or you simply feel like it or for any other reason. Having to eat regularly to remain energized and active is nothing but a myth. The fear of entering 'starvation mode' looms so large that we end up eating far more than what we need.

Our body is well-equipped to manage not just missing a couple of meals but times of great famine. So, if you do not feel hungry, don't hesitate to skip a couple of meals. Just be conscious of not overeating when you do sit down to your meal after a couple of skips. Also, stick to healthy foods during your meal times. The trick in intermittent fasting is to cut calorie intake by cutting down the number of meals.

Skipping meals whenever you feel inclined is referred to as spontaneous intermitting fasting. The flipside of this method is a lack of plan and strategy that could lead you to become irreverent and undisciplined in your approach leading to ineffective results. However, if you are a naturally disciplined person and have ingrained the habit of intermittent fasting into your system, then the spontaneous method will work perfectly.

Fundamental Pros and Cons of Intermittent Fasting

While the detailed benefits and cautions to take while on intermittent are discussed in Chapter 4 and 5, this is a good place to give you some fundamental and obvious pros and cons of intermittent fasting, and these hold good irrespective of the type of IF you choose to go with.

The Positives of Intermittent Fasting

If you plan your meals to fit into a smaller eating window, you are more likely to be a conscious eater than if you choose to leave the entire day open to eat whenever you like. With intermittent fasting, you tend to become a more mindful eater than before. Eating mindlessly is one of the biggest causes of binge-eating (discussed in Chapter 7).

Another thing about intermittent fasting is that while you have to keep a general control over calorie intake, you don't have to micromanage this aspect. Therefore, given the freedom to eat what you want (in reasonable amounts) could actually drive you to consume healthier foods. Many times, excessive restrictions drive us to do something we should not do. Intermittent fasting gives you a reasonable amount of freedom to eat your favorite foods during your eating window.

The Negatives of Intermittent Fasting

For some people, the fact that you can eat whatever you want can be counterproductive because they end up binge-eating at every meal during the eating window. This approach will end up defeating the core desire of intermittent fasting and you could eat far more than needed resulting in weight gain and an unhealthy lifestyle.

The initial hiccups could drive some people to overreact to hunger pangs and cravings resulting in cultivating worse eating habits than before. All the initial setbacks of intermittent fasting and how to cope with them are discussed in Chapter 6 in greater detail.

Moreover, restricting the time of eating could also make some people think that it is another form of 'diet.' This dieting mindset can be detrimental to achieving your intermittent fasting goals. A compulsive mindset of 'following a diet' will make you less likely to follow through the process than you look at it as an altered eating pattern.

The most important thing you must remember about intermittent fasting is that it is not some crash diet that you can try for 3-5 days before an upcoming party to fit into a dress you've bought for yourself. It is a choice of a lifetime to change the way you eat for the rest of your life.

Read on for more benefits, cautionary advice, and more

about intermittent fasting.

Chapter 4

Benefits of Intermittent Fasting

Numerous studies prove and reiterate the multiple benefits of intermittent fasting leveraged by our ancestors knowingly or unknowingly. Intermittent fasting has positive effects both on your body and mind. When you start your regimen, you will notice many good things taking place in your body. Let us look at some of the benefits of intermittent fasting.

Intermittent Fasting and Weight Loss

The primary reason why intermittent fasting helps you lose weight is that you automatically consume fewer calories. Every type of intermittent fasting consists of skipping one or two meals during the fasting window. Unless you overeat unnecessarily during the eating window, in effect, you are reducing your calorie intake significantly.

Intermittent fasting is a preferred choice over many fad

diets for weight loss because you do not need to spend resources on measuring and managing your food consumption in an annoyingly meticulous way. You don't really need to track your calorie and nutrient intake from the meals you consume during the eating window.

Intermittent fasting forces your body to reach out to its own fat reserves because you are depriving it of immediate energy fuel by not eating. By cutting down your food intake, your body does not have access to 'easy' glucose, and therefore, has no option but to delve into its fat reserves for its fuel needs.

Multiple studies and surveys have revealed intermittent fasting reduced body weight by 3% - 8% over a period of 3-24 weeks. The alternate-day fasting method helped volunteers lose an average of 0.75 pounds per week as against the other methods of intermittent fasting which resulted in an average per-week weight loss of 0.55 pounds.

People on intermittent fasting also lost 4-7% from their waistline which revealed loss of belly fat too. These impressive results were not of one or two studies but multiple studies conducted over a period of time across the globe. Moreover, all these studies also revealed that intermittent fasting led to fat loss and not lean muscle loss.

So, here is a little summary of how fasting and fat burning is connected:

- It takes at least 12 hours of fasting before any significant amount of fat is burned for fuel.

- The longer the fasting period, the more of the fat reserves are used up for fuel.

- Being active (working normally or going for a walk) during your fasting period can increase the amount of fat that is being burned; however, excessive physical training, running marathons, etc. should not be done.

- Some people's metabolism is more flexible than others' which means they get into a fat-burning state much faster and more effectively. The good thing here is that with a few weeks of intermittent fasting practice, it is possible to increase your metabolic flexibility too.

Factors to Keep in Mind for Weight Loss

A critical point to note is weight loss with intermittent fasting will happen effectively only when you maintain a calorie deficiency. Here are a couple of useful pointers:

Food quality – Stick to nutritious, natural, whole-grained, and fiber-rich foods while avoiding junk and processed foods

Calories – If you choose to overeat during the eating window and 'compensate' for the loss of calories during the fasting window, you will not get the benefit of weight loss. During your eating window, eat as if you did not fast just before that time.

Consistency – Intermittent fasting does not work like a fly-by-night profit-making shell company. It is a solid global enterprise that is here to stay and, therefore, will take time to show its excellent results. Be consistent with your efforts over a sustained period of time for effective weight loss results.

Patience – Again, intermittent fasting is not a magic trick. It uses and leverages the body's natural mechanism to reach out to available alternate fuel sources (primarily, fat). Your body is bound to resist changes you are trying to bring about, and it will take time for it to adjust to these changes. Be patient, persist in your efforts, and wait for the adjustment period to finish before expecting results.

Exercise – Intermittent fasting does not give you the liberty to remain physically inactive. You have to continue with your exercise regimen for optimal weight loss benefits. In fact, some studies have proven exercising on an empty stomach have plenty of fitness and health benefits.

Exercising and fasting optimize cellular factors that affect fat metabolism positively resulting in faster and more effective weight loss than if you used only one of the two. However, there are some counter-indications for women, especially on the aspect of reproductive capabilities. Fasting and women is a topic that is dealt with in a bit of detail in Chapter 6.

Health Benefits

Maintains healthy blood sugar levels

Carbohydrates from the food we eat is broken down into glucose or sugar in our bloodstream. Insulin transports the glucose from our bloodstream to the cells where it is converted into energy. Diabetes is a condition in which insulin does not function effectively leading to high levels of sugar in the bloodstream along with multiple symptoms such as frequent urination, thirst, and fatigue.

Studies on intermittent fasting eating patterns have proved that it helps in maintaining blood sugar levels by preventing insulin, sugar spikes and crashes leading to reduced risks of diabetes. Other studies were conducted with participants who had diabetes, and the observations from these studies revealed intermittent fasting not only helped in weight loss and control calorie intake but also reduced blood sugar levels.

Studies also proved that individuals on intermittent fasting eating patterns showed a 12% decrease in blood sugar level and 53% reduction in insulin levels. These figures are reflective of the power of intermittent fasting methods in maintaining healthy blood sugar levels. Lowered insulin levels in the bloodstream prevent build-up which, in turn, increases our insulin-sensitivity allowing the critical hormone to work more efficiently.

Improves Heart Health

Intermittent fasting is proven to have a lot of benefits for heart health by lowering incidences of certain heart-related risk factors or health markers as they are known in medical terminology.

Studies proved that intermittent fasting reduces unhealthy triglycerides and LDL cholesterol levels and increases healthy HDL cholesterol levels. In some intermittent fasting studies on animals, it was observed that adiponectin protein levels improved. This protein involved in the metabolism of sugar and fat is believed to be useful in the prevention of heart attacks and heart disorders.

Intermittent fasting is also known to balance blood pressure levels, another key risk factor for heart problems. Although many of these studies are animal-based, experts are of the opinion that these benefits could be manifested in humans too.

Reduces Inflammation and Oxidative Stress

Although inflammation is nothing but our body's natural immune response to any kind of injury, chronic inflammation can potentially cause health disorders. Some studies, in fact, have connected chronic inflammation to cancer, heart disease, obesity, and diabetes.

Studies on people who were following the Ramadan fast showed reduced levels of inflammatory-related risk factors. Nighttime fasts were also linked to lowered levels of inflammatory markers. Alternate-day fasting studies revealed lowered risk factors associated with oxidative stress, another marker directly connected to risks of chronic diseases.

Oxidation is a process that involves free radicals, or unstable molecules, to react with and damage healthy and stable molecules such as proteins and DNA. Multiple studies have revealed the usefulness of intermittent fasting to build our resistance to oxidative stress.

Improves Brain Function and Cognitive Abilities and Reduces Neurodegenerative Risks

Most elements that are good for your body are typically good for the brain too, and so it is with intermittent fasting. Intermittent fasting is shown to improve multiple metabolic features critical for the health of your brain and for improved cognitive functions.

These metabolic features that get a boost with intermittent fasting include reduced inflammation, oxidative stress, reduced blood sugar levels, and improved insulin sensitivity. Some animal studies have revealed that intermittent fasting can help in the growth of new nerve cells which could have a direct connection to brain function.

Additionally, intermittent fasting is believed to improve levels of brain-derived neurotrophic factor (BDNF), an important brain hormone. BDNF is a protein which interacts with the nerve cells in the basal forebrain, hippocampus, and cortex; all of which are linked to human cognitive functions such as learning and memory.

BDNF is also known to facilitate the survival and growth of existing neurons as well as stimulating the growth of new neurons. It is also connected to the neuro-synaptic connectivity between neurons. The deficiency of this critical brain hormone is connected to depression and other brain-related mental disorders including cognitive impairment, memory loss, and Alzheimer's. In fact, antidepressants increase the level of BDNF, and so does fasting.

Animal studies have also revealed that intermittent fasting could protect the brain from stroke-related damage. Intermittent fasting studies on animals have also revealed that it could delay the onset or reduce the symptoms of neurodegenerative diseases such as Alzheimer's, Huntington's, and Parkinson's.

Healthy Pancreas and Liver

The pancreas is the organ responsible for the production and release of insulin. As your body becomes more sensitive to insulin, the pancreas does not get overworked by overproduction of this critical hormone leading to a healthy pancreas.

Intermittent fasting is also known to make your liver healthy by helping it fight against excessive storage of fat. Intermittent fasting produces proteins responsible for the absorption and storage of fatty acids in the liver thereby freeing it from having to absorb and hold too much fat.

Improved Sensitivity to Hunger Cues

Leptin, produced by fat cells, is a hormone connected to satiety. It sends signals to you to stop eating when satiated. Leptin levels increase when you feel full and decrease when you feel hungry.

As fat cells produce leptin, obese and overweight individuals typically have high levels of leptin in their body. Excessive leptin potentially leads to leptin resistance thereby making it difficult for your body to read and turn off hunger cues when you are feeling full.

Studies conducted on people who were following intermittent fasting revealed lower levels of leptin during the fasting period. Reduced leptin levels typically translate to improved leptin sensitivity enabling your body to interpret hunger cues well and prevent overeating.

Intermittent fasting helps in correcting eating disorders by enhancing the body's sensitivity to the various hormones. It helps in reversing binge eating and resetting the natural eating pattern of the human body.

Improves Lifespan

Intermittent fasting studies on animals have revealed its ability to extend lifespan. Many of the studies on rats gave startling results wherein the rats that were on alternate-day fasting lived 83% longer than those animals which were not on any fast.

Other Healthy Changes in Your Body

Improved Productivity and Energy

When we consume excessive foods, especially processed foods, our minds become dull and our energies are at a low level. On the contrary, studies have proven that on an empty stomach, focus and concentration powers improve significantly.

When you fast, the energies that would have been used to digest the consumed food will be channelized for other more productive work including cell repair and regeneration. Additionally, enhanced cognitive powers (a benefit of intermittent fasting) also help in improving alertness, focus, and mental accuracy.

Fasting makes you feel 'light' which gives you an energy boost. Another reason for this boost of energy is that during a normal eating pattern, our energy source is from carbs and sugars which provide 4 calories per gram. When on a fasting pattern, your body draws energy from fats which give 9 calories per gram thereby boosting our natural energy levels.

Improved Skin Texture

Oxidative stress from free radicals and chronic inflammation can damage and cause your skin to wrinkle up and form fine lines as well. Intermittent fasting reduces both oxidative stress and inflammation resulting in improved and smooth skin texture. Intermittent fasting helps clear your skin of acne and pimples giving it a glowing, vibrant look.

Improved Lean Mass

During any weight loss program, you would typically lose both muscle and fat. Losing fat is great but losing muscle is not. Intermittent fasting speeds up fat metabolism resulting in more fat loss and insignificant lean mass loss.

Flatter belly

When the body turns to fat for its fuel, it succeeds in breaking down and releasing energy from stubborn belly fat too. Therefore, a sustained effort at intermittent fasting is bound to help you achieve a flatter belly than before.

Improved Motor Skills

Motor abilities such balancing can be affected significantly with aging. There are multiple studies which prove that improved fasting helps in decreasing the effects of motor disabilities associated with aging.

Improved Sleep

Research studies have proven that intermittent fasting can improve sleeping patterns and can reset your sleeping pattern if it has been disturbed by travel.

Improved Sensitivity to Taste

Getting addicted to excessively sugary, salty, and processed foods is easy. However, the overwhelming tastes from these types of foods lower our taste buds' sensitivity. The taste buds forget how to appreciate and savor wholesome, earthy, and healthy flavors.

After a fasting period, your taste buds are reset to the original natural state, and these grainy and earthy flavors become delicious again. Moreover, as you sustain your fasting efforts, you will notice that you will lessen the amounts of sugars and salts in your food to savor their taste. Even the subtlest of flavors are easily discernible by your sensitive taste buds.

Psychological Benefits

In addition to physical and other health benefits that fasting offers, there is a multitude of psychological benefits you can take advantage of when you choose the intermittent fasting way of staying healthy and fit. Let's explore some of these psychological benefits.

Improved Willpower

Sabotaging behaviors, destructive addictions, and giving

in to your desires without a fight are all examples of the opposite of willpower. All these elements slowly but surely ruin your life and relationships. Bad decisions taken because of the lack of willpower will weaken you even further and stunt your growth and development.

If you continue to justify your poor decisions because of your weak willpower, you are only adding fuel to the fire, creating irreparable bad habits for life. Bad habits are a reflection of your inability to control yourself, and if you cannot control yourself, you can hardly control anything else.

Fasting is a natural way of learning to control your responses and reactions to your physical needs and desires. When you fast, you are voluntarily choosing not to eat, even under the pressure of hunger pangs. You are choosing to fast (give up food) to gain something else (health and fitness).

Food is the most basic element of survival, and eating when hungry is the fundamental survival instinct. Therefore, when you control this basic survival instinct by choosing not to eat even when you feel hungry, you will find your willpower increasing in strength. You will find the power to control other less fundamental and yet, debilitating bad habits that are ruining your life.

Fasting is the most natural and the most sophisticated form of workout to build your willpower. If you develop the habit of fasting, you will be able to control many other debilitating habits of your life more efficiently. In fact, there are medical studies which prove that fasting can dissipate cravings for alcohol, nicotine, caffeine, etc.

So, build and strengthen your willpower by making intermittent fasting a habit in your life.

Improves Self-Confidence

Self-control is the foundation of self-confidence. Confidence is nothing but a reflection of your ability for self-control. So, when you lose self-control, you are effectively sabotaging your self-confidence. The reverse is also true. When you build your self-control, you build and strengthen your self-confidence.

Lack of self-confidence causes plenty of internal conflicts which have the debilitating power of corroding your willpower. These unceasing internal conflicts leave you exhausted and on a perpetual defensive mode resulting in further reduction in self-confidence.

Now, suppose you build your self-control and behave the way you always intended to behave. The results of these intended actions will build your self-confidence as you develop greater trust in your capabilities and strengths. With each success, you will find the power to take on more challenging goals and tasks and eventually build your self-efficacy to such an extent that you are in complete control of your future and destiny.

Fasting is the most effective way to practice self-control and, consequently build self-confidence. Medical studies have also revealed that fasting improves catecholamines in your body. Catecholamines (for example, dopamine) are believed to be connected to your happiness, confidence, and feel-good emotions and also reduce anxiety and stress levels.

Improved Clarity of Thought

With enhanced brain functioning and cognitive powers, your ability to think clearly will improve. Eating dulls your thoughts and fasting creates clarity. When you fast, your brain and body are able to catch even subtle signals and you can see the things going wrong in your life.

While fasting, you can very quickly notice the incongruent elements in your life such as bad habits, poor organization, lack of purpose and intention, and more. This clear perspective is bound to make you take corrective steps.

With improved willpower and self-confidence, you will find the necessary physical and mental strength to overcome challenges and improve the overall quality of your life. Fasting can be a great resetting mode for the psychological aspect of your life.

Improved Emotions

Excessive eating is effectively an emotional dependency. Foods such as processed sugars, caffeine, and trans-fatty acids, and alcohol are all known to over-stimulate our emotions and, therefore, abstaining from eating occasionally helps in stabilizing our emotions.

Fasting can also reset your negative emotion pattern and you can break free of their harmful effects. Moreover, fasting helps us have a different perceptive of our environment enhancing our clarity to see what and how things are going wrong in our lives. Such sharp perceptions automatically drive us to reshape our environments for improved quality of life.

The sustained efforts of intermittent fasting can have startling benefits for you. Each one of the benefits mentioned in this chapter are possible. Some of them may manifest faster than others. Patience, perseverance, and commitment are vital elements to leverage nearly all the benefits of intermittent fasting.

Chapter 5

What to Expect in the Initial Days

There is no doubt that fasting is a powerful tool for weight loss and healthy living. However, there are certain things that you must prepare yourself for before you start off on your intermittent fasting journey.

Things to Know and Do Before You Start Intermittent Fasting

One of the first things you must know before you take your step is that if you have been consuming foods irregularly and without focusing on quality of nutrients, then you will have more challenges as compared to someone who has been eating nutrient-rich foods. Only when you change the quality of food, will fasting have the necessary beneficial effects on your body and mind.

The second most important thing is if you are consistently going to eat processed carb-rich foods in your eating window, then too, losing weight or staying healthy will not work even if you fast.

Therefore, work out your meal plans for your eating window, and stick to home-cooked meals prepared with fresh, organic ingredients. Stock up on good-quality ingredients at home. Look at Chapter 8 for useful tips on what to eat and what to avoid.

Decide which meal you plan to skip, and stick to this decision, at least until your body has got accustomed to the routine. Later on, you can change the meal you wish to skip depending on your dynamic lifestyle. However, initially, make a choice at the beginning itself, and don't waver from it.

So, for example, if you have chosen to skip breakfast in the 16:8 intermittent fasting method, then eat your lunch at the usual time you eat. Slowly, as your body gets used to the new eating pattern, you can shift your lunchtime by an hour or two taking your fasting window to 18 instead of 16 hours.

Planning is essential for effective benefits. You have to spend time and energy prepping so that fresh and wholesome meals are kept handy and ready for your eating window. Without proper preparation and planning, you are bound to eat foods that should be avoided thereby losing out on the benefits. It is imperative you keep your body amply hydrated when you fast because you will not be getting water from food.

Expected Side Effects and How to Cope With Them

When you alter your eating pattern, expect a transition period which is going to be tough. However, this transition period is temporary, and when your body gets used to the new eating pattern, all the benefits will manifest, and you will feel an amazing sense of achievement in addition to feeling lighter and healthier than before. Therefore, expect and accept the transition period.

One way of looking at the transition period is to remind yourself that you are not starving. You are only choosing not to eat for your own good. Despite these nice-sounding (and true) words, you will undergo some unpleasant side-effects in the initial days. Here are some side-effects of intermittent fasting along with a few tips on how to overcome them:

Hunger Pangs

Your body has gotten used to receiving 4-5 meals a day, and suddenly when you turn off that tap, it is going to rebel because it expects those meals to come at the fixed times that it has gotten accustomed to.

Remember that hormone, leptin, that switches on and off the hunger cues? When you were overeating, your body was filled with that hormone and you could never get the correct hunger cues from it. Now, that you have started fasting, your body will become sensitive to the presence of leptin, and send signals to your brain when you feel hungry triggering symptoms of hunger.

Moreover, when you were on a normal diet, the hunger hormone would peak at breakfast, lunch, and dinner times. This pattern will continue until your body understands that it is not going to get food as before.

Fighting off hunger pangs can be a huge challenge in the initial days of your fasting, and it will take an immense amount of willpower to win against it. Three to five days into your regimen will be the worst days. If you can survive these initial few days, you will be fine. In fact, soon you will begin to notice that the eating window has already started and you are not feeling as hungry as when you first started.

The best way to combat hunger pangs in the initial days of intermittent fasting is by hydrating your body with plenty of plain water. A belly full of water will prevent you from responding to the urge of putting something into your mouth. Drink small amounts of water frequently.

Intermittent fasting will also teach you to discern between feeling thirsty and feeling hungry clearly. Moreover, you will realize that before your intermittent fasting days, you were eating more often than needed to stave off boredom.

More Tips to Stave off Hunger Pangs

Understand the Difference Between Physical and Emotional Hunger - Yes, hunger pangs are real and you need to manage them. However, know the difference between physical and psychological or emotional hunger pangs. Here are some tips to differentiate between the two types of hunger pangs:

- Physical hunger comes gradually and can be easily postponed. Emotional hunger comes on suddenly and without reason and is very difficult to postpone.

- Physical hunger can be satiated with any kind of food. Emotional hunger can be satiated only with specific cravings such as ice-cream, chocolate, pizzas, etc.

- When you eat because of physical hunger, you can easily stop eating when you are full. Emotional hunger pangs drive you to eat more than needed leaving you feeling uncomfortably full.

- When physical hunger is appeased, you feel satisfied, and not guilty. Emotional hunger pangs only result in feelings of guilt.

Many times, when we 'feel' hungry, it is not physical hunger but emotional hunger. Once we understand the difference, then we can manage our eating patterns much better. A little bit of unwiring in the head will free us from our emotional hunger pangs and prevent us from excessive eating.

Balance Your Macronutrients in Every Meal – Make sure you get sufficient quantities of carbs, proteins, and fats at every meal to prevent hunger pangs setting in sooner than needed.

Don't Mistake Thirst for Hunger – Many times, just a drink of water will make us feel better because we mistake thirst for hunger. Drink lots of water to prevent hunger pangs.

Try tea and coffee – Green tea is the best option. However, black and sugarless coffee and tea can also help you manage hunger. You have many flavored teas (chocolate, strawberry, coconut) for added comfort.

Try chewing gum – Again, ensure you use sugarless gums. Chewing gum takes your mind off hunger.

Eat a teaspoon of psyllium husk – This fiber-rich supplement is a great zero-calorie ingredient that can signal your brain into thinking food has been supplied to the body and reduce the feeling of hunger.

Brush your teeth – This activity has known to stave off hunger, perhaps, because of the flavor of the toothpaste.

Keep busy and active – Indulge in an activity that will make you forget hunger. If you are a working professional, then that itself will take care of it. You will have no time to feel hungry, especially the emotional hunger. When you are in the flow of an activity, you will never realize how fast 4-6 hours will fly, and this is the time needed to reach the 16- or 18-hour fasting duration.

Cravings

When you don't eat for a long time, your mind will continuously dwell on food and related topics. You are bound to be thinking of food unwittingly because of the hunger pangs. Moreover, when your body is starved of glucose (which is what happens during fasting), you will crave for all the wrong kinds of foods including refined carbohydrates and sweets.

These cravings, though only temporary, can break your routine even before your body gets used to the intermittent schedule. Managing them during the initial stages will help you get into your fasting schedule more easily than if you gave in to them. Find ways to prevent overthinking about food. Here are tips on how to overcome food cravings during your fasting window.

Sleep well – When your body is altering its routine, it's

important not to add stress by reducing your sleep. In the initial days of your intermittent fasting, ensure you get your daily dose of sleep. Lack of restful sleep can enhance feelings of hunger and cravings.

Eat your meals at the scheduled times during your eating window – You will not forget the first meal after your fasting window ends because hunger pangs would have set in. You must also remember not to forget the 2nd or 3rd meal that you have planned. If you forget and your fasting window begins, then your body has not had a sufficient dosage of nutrition and is bound to set in the cravings scene earlier.

Include your cravings into your diet plan – For example, if you need that sweet, include a small bowl of fruit with yogurt in your meals. If you are craving salt, plan a spicy wholegrain sandwich as part of your scheduled meal. Do not eat it as a separate snack during the fasting window. Convince yourself that the cravings will be satiated during the eating window.

Maintain a journal of your cravings – While this will not physically stop your cravings, looking at the list of foods you are craving and the needless calories it will add to your system can be a powerful deterrent to consuming it. Moreover, this journal will help you understand your craving cycle and identify the peak times so that you can manage them prudently. It will also help you identify craving triggers.

Eat varied meals – A variety of foods on your plate will take care of multiple cravings. Don't stick to one kind of dish. Include fruit and vegetables, try new combinations, include a favorite drink, and more such variety. Meals with varied dishes will help you manage cravings well.

Make sure every meal in your eating window has sufficient macronutrients. If you don't give your body sufficient carbohydrates, proteins, and fats, the cravings will hit you sooner and harder than otherwise. Make sure most of your calories are from your macronutrients consumed through wholesome and fresh ingredients.

Headaches

Your body is being subjected to new changes, and headaches are a common way of making you aware of its resistance to the changes you are imposing on it. Here are some tips to manage headaches during intermittent fasting:

Stay hydrated - Hydration is one of the most useful ways of managing these headaches. The lack of sufficient water in your body could be a trigger for headaches. Ensure you drink plenty of water during your eating and fasting windows.

Protect your sense organs – Your body is already under some amount of stress because of the lack of food. Don't add to this stress by exposing yourself and your sense organs to excessive headache stimulants such as loud noises, powerful smells, and flashing lights. Wear earplugs to block out annoying noises. Put some peppermint oil under your nose to keep you from unpleasant smells. Wear sunglasses when you know you are going to be exposed to a lot of lights.

Avoid stress and other triggers – During your fasting schedule, avoid meeting with people that add stress to your life. Keep your difficult appointments and tasks for the eating window. Relax your body and mind through meditation or yoga or by simply indulging in your favorite hobby.

Headaches triggered by fasting are temporary and will disappear once your body gets accustomed to the new eating schedule.

Low Energy – Your body is suddenly being deprived of its regular source of energy which is consumption of food 3-4 times a day. So, initially, it will feel like you don't have the energy to do a lot of activities. Keep your day as relaxed as possible so that you can conserve energy.

Align your fitness regime with your eating schedule. In fact, until the intermittent fasting schedule has set in, it might make sense to cut out your strenuous workouts and stick to simple physical activities such as walking or yoga.

Once your body recognizes the fat sources and gets

accustomed to drawing energy from its fat reserves, the energy level will actually see a huge improvement. Fat gives 9 calories per gm!

Constipation, Heartburn, and Bloating –
Your digestive system produces acid for the digestive process, and when you don't eat, this acid could cause some mild heartburn in some people. Depending on your constitution, this could range from very mild to a full-time painful experience.

Typically, time is an excellent cure for this temporary side effect because it will disappear with time. Sufficient hydration, avoiding spicy, fried, and other foods that enhance heartburn effects and other simple activities will take care of it. If the heartburn persists, don't hesitate to visit your physician.

Intermittent fasting could also result in constipation which, in turn, could give you a bloating, gassy feeling. Drinking water and waiting out for the symptoms to go away works best.

Irritability – Hunger pangs are real. They are not imaginary. Your body is telling you it needs the food you were routinely giving it. These hunger pangs combined with crazy cravings will enhance your irritability levels and you will notice you are losing your temper far more frequently than before. This is a very personal emotion and you will have to manage it the best way you can.

One is to tell your loved ones and close colleagues that you have started intermittent fasting. Most people will understand and cut you some slack. Second, avoid difficult situations as much as you can during the fasting window. Focus on doing things that make you happy.

Feeling Cold – Feeling cold, especially in your hands and feet, is a common side-effect of intermittent fasting. This sense of coldness is a very good thing and has a very simple explanation. When you fast, your body increased blood flow (referred to as adipose tissue blood flow) to its fat reserves. This increased amount of blood is a sign that your fat reserves are being used up for energy which is what intermittent fasting wants to achieve. Additionally, reduced levels of blood sugar make us feel more sensitive to cold.

Wear warm clothing, sip hot tea, take warm showers, and indulge in non-calorific activities to reduce the coldness. Also, avoid being out in the cold for prolonged periods of time.

Overeating – This is the first side-effect that you must be conscious of and avoid right from the beginning. Excessive consumption of food during the eating window is the most common reason for intermittent fasting to fail. There are many reasons why you tend to overeat in the initial days of intermittent fasting:

- Cravings and hunger pangs reach their peaks and we end up eating to satiate these cravings and not for nutrition.

- The overexcitement of eating food after a fasting window drives us to go overboard.

- A misconception that intermittent fasting does not require counting calories.

Overeating during the eating window beats the very purpose of using intermittent fasting for weight loss and a healthy life. It is important to be wary of this side-effect and plan your meals so that you don't overeat. Here are some tips for meal planning and prep work and a few cooking hacks so that you eat healthy, nutritious food during the eating window.

Set aside time and energy for meal planning and prep – Meal planning and prep is an important activity for the success of your intermittent fasting, and therefore, you must commit yourself to spend the necessary time and energy towards this critical activity. It might make sense to set aside this planning and prep activity for the weekend, perhaps the Saturday afternoon or Sunday morning.

However, you can choose the time based on your lifestyle and working schedules. If you think, spending a little time every day for the next day's meal plan and prep, then go ahead. Just remember not to ignore this crucial activity of intermittent fasting.

Plan your grocery shopping in advance –
For this, you must first sit down and decide what meals
you will eat during the week, and then buy the grocery
aligning with your weekly meal plan.

**Read, learn, and memorize the calories of
the macronutrients in your food** – Initially,
this might be a little tough and could take up a lot of
time. However, as you persist, within a few weeks, you
will notice you can rattle off calorie values of nearly all
macronutrients in your diet. Knowing your calorie
numbers well, you can plan your meals to match your
needs. Take care of portion sizes while keeping track of
calories.

Be realistic – Don't overdo the planning and try to
achieve perfection in trying to get every meal and every
snack ready beforehand. If you do take this approach,
you might be adding undue stress to an already stressed
out body system. Take things slowly, accept
imperfections in your planning process as being normal,
learn as you progress, and simply don't give up because
of temporary setbacks.

**Avoid being overly creative with your
foods** – Again, focusing on creativity during the initial
stages of your intermittent fasting time can be more
stressful than needed. Avoid it and keep your meal plans
simple and easy. Once your body and mind have adjusted
to intermittent fasting, then you can give wings to your
creativity. Until then, rein in.

Learn smart and easy ways of cooking – There are a lot of prepping hacks you can learn and use. Buy chopped and frozen vegetables. Pick up recipes that need just one cook; put everything inside and turn on the heat, and wait for the cooking to finish. Make two or three batches of dishes and freeze them for a couple of days and save cooking time. Always choose the easy way out instead of overcomplicating things, resulting in overeating when you shouldn't.

Take breaks during your meal – After you have eaten half of your planned meal, take a 10-minute break, and check if you are still feeling hungry. Only if you are absolutely sure that you need more food, then resume your meal. Else, refrigerate the leftover for the next meal. Remember to stop eating when your stomach is 3/4ths full.

A Lot More Trips to the Bathroom

Remember you are drinking more water than you used to. Increased hydration will increase the number of trips to the bathroom. There is no way to avoid these trips, and in fact, avoiding them could be harmful. Each visit to the bathroom is removing more toxins from your body, and so, bathroom trips are good.

The side-effects mentioned above might make you feel that intermittent fasting is tough. Well, that is not true at all. All these side-effects are only temporary, and typically, will disappear in a week or so. One of the best ways to keep these side-effects to the minimum is to ease yourself into intermittent fasting slowly. Don't jump to the 18:6 method on the first day. Start with the 12:12 method, prepare yourself for the preparatory work, and as you gain confidence, enhance the fasting window gradually.

Finally, always, always listen to what your body is telling you. Each of us is unique and some of us could find it easy, others not so easy, and while still others may never be able to use this method. Pay attention to your body and the cues it is giving you and respond appropriately.

How to Track Progress

Checking your weight once a week is the most common way people check their progress. However, checking your weight alone is not enough because body weight can vary up to 2 kg up or down without any internal changes in your body. These random variations in weight make it difficult to see the right kind of progress based only in the weighing scale reading. Other factors also have to be tracked to see if your intermittent fasting journey is on the right track. Let us look at some of these important factors.

Measure Your Waist

Visceral fat is the fat that sits around your internal organs resulting in a huge belly. Visceral fat is the biggest contributors of ill-health and low levels of fitness. Studies have proven that a big belly resulting from excessive visceral fat increases risks of diabetes, heart diseases, and other cardiovascular disorders. The fat under your bottom, skin, lower abdomen and thighs are believed to be far less harmful than belly fat.

Ideally, your belly must be less than half your height. Some studies prove that individuals with normal BMI have excessive belly fat. In such cases, it is possible to be misled by the 'normal' BMI and forget about the more dangerous belly fat. Intermittent fasting is known to be one of the best ways to lose risk-enhancing visceral fat. So, if you are looking to lose weight for improving your health, you must track your visceral fat by measuring your belly or waist.

Now, which part of your belly will give you the correct measurement of your waist? Well, the natural waist comes approximately halfway between the navel and the ribs. This is the best place to measure your waistline. Don't pull the tape tight. Just let it rest upon your skin. If you must suck in your breath, remember you can do it only once. Just make sure it is at the same level for each measure. This technique will give you a good idea of the measure of your waist.

Check Your Weight

While most training centers and gyms have a mechanism of checking your weight once a week, it may not give you the most accurate result of your weight loss progress. The most effective way to check your weight is to weigh yourself every day, and take an average once every ten days or a fortnight. There are valid reasons why checking your weight once a week will not give accurate figures.

The amount of water your body holds varies significantly. For example, if you have eaten carb-rich or salty foods, then your body retains a lot more water than you have eaten foods with less salt and fewer carbs. When you weigh yourself every day, you will easily see the connection between an increased reading and your salt/carb intake. In fact, there are times when your body weight will show an increase of nearly 1 kg if you have eaten a lot of carb-rich and/or salt-rich food, perhaps, on a non-fasting day.

Hormonal changes and regular muscle damage brought on by exercising and training also make your body retain water, resulting in increased weight. All these weight gains are not 'real' gains and are not brought on by the accumulation of fat.

Fasting, on the other hand, drives your body to lose water to use the stored glycogen. So, in the initial days of your intermittent fasting, your weight could drop significantly. However, these are not 'fat losses' and, therefore, do not reflect 'real' weight loss. Therefore, weight checks done only once a week will not give you accurate results because on the day you weighed yourself, you will not know if the weight gain or loss is real or not. The more accurate way is to weigh yourself daily, and then, take an average regularly.

Another effective way of checking your weight progress is to do it once a month instead of daily or weekly. A month is a sufficiently long period for real fat losses to reflect on your body weight. Ideally, people on intermittent fasting lose about 2 kg per month. Some pointers regarding weight checks:

- It is needless to panic about fluctuations in your weight. These fluctuations are normal.

- Weigh yourself every day and take an average.

- Alternately, check your weight once a month.

- Look at the general trend in your weight loss. If you have lost 2 kg in the first 2 weeks and then there is no movement in the downward direction for the next two weeks, the average weight loss for 4 weeks is 2 kg which is the ideal target for intermittent fasters.

- Weigh yourself at the same time each day wearing similar clothing. The ideal time is in the morning after you wake up and finished your bathroom trip.

- If you are a panicky kind of person, then stick to the monthly regimen instead of daily.

Remember, weight loss is not a smooth, seamless, and steady process. It is full of ups and downs which can be brought on by many factors beyond your control too. So, don't panic. Choose and stick to one regimen of measuring your weight.

Measure your body fat

Weight loss is effectively achieved by fat loss. Therefore, it makes sense to measure your body fat instead of (or in addition to) your body weight. There are good and reasonably priced body fat analyzers that are available in the market; either as part of a weighing scale or a separate device. It would be a worthwhile investment for you and others in your family.

While the readings of these devices might not be accurate to the last gram of fat, it will give you a general trend of whether your body fat is increasing or decreasing which is good enough to see if your intermittent fasting is moving on the right track or not.

The principle of a body fat analyzer is based on the fact that an electrical impulse moves faster through water than through fat. So, a tiny electrical impulse is run through your body and its speed is calculated by the machine. This speed is used to determine the fat as a percentage of the body weight.

Considering that it is a percentage figure if your body has retained or lost more water because of the reasons already discussed under **Check Your Weight**, then the fat reading will be inaccurate just like your body weight reading. Therefore, here too, it is sensible to average our daily readings, or better still, measure your body fat only once a month. The same conditions of body weight measure hold good for body fat measure too.

Other Tracking Methods

In addition to weight, fat content, and other visible aspects of progress, there are multiple health benefits which can be used to track your progress in the intermittent fasting journey. Here are some of these health benefits:

Blood Pressure

Studies have proved that even a small percentage drop (5-10%) in overall weight can reduce blood pressure (BP) readings too. Therefore, you can employ your BP readings to see how you are progressing. However, a random BP check done when you visit your physician will not give you an accurate representation of progress.

You must monitor BP readings at home using highly affordable blood monitors available on the market. The best time to read your BP is in the morning and in the evening. Typically, your BP starts to rise when you wake up, continues to rise as the day progresses, and begins to fall again during the evening. Tips to read your BP:

- You must be in a relaxed frame of mind, sitting comfortably, and feeling sufficiently warm.

- You should not have eaten or exercised at least an hour before you check your BP.

- The BP monitor should be at the same level as your heart as you take your readings.

- Make sure you follow the instructions given in the manual that comes along with the BP monitor.

- You must take three readings with a few minutes gap between each reading.

- Ignore the first one, and take the average of the second and the third reading; the first is more to get your body and mind ready for the reading.

- An ideal BP reading is 119/70. However, anything less than 140/90 is fine.

Glucose Tolerance

The blood sugar levels tested before a meal (fasting) and at a prescribed time after a meal will give you your glucose tolerance. You can measure this at your physician's office or blood-sugar monitors for home use are available at affordable rates on the market. A normal fasting reading is between 70 mg/dL and 100 mg/dL. If your readings are consistently between 110 and 135, then there is an increased risk of diabetes. If your readings are reducing, then your intermittent fasting is on track.

Other tests including blood cholesterol and IGF-1 (insulin-like growth hormone) will also give you a good indication of your progress. These tests, however, have to be done at your physician's office only.

Chapter 6

Intermittent Fasting Is Not

For All

Intermittent fasting, as you might already know, is an age-old practice that has found a lot of scientific backing in the modern times. Research studies have proved the efficacy of intermittent fasting in preventing multiple health disorders, all of which have been discussed in Chapter 3.

Yes, it is excellent for people for whom it is suitable which includes nearly everyone. You can lose fat, gain lean mass, and manage to consume all important nutrients without excessive calories getting into your system.

However, random skipping of meals while overeating in other meals will not achieve what you set out to. In addition to skipping meals, you must pay attention to nutritional specifics so that you get the best out of the eating pattern.

Intermittent fasting, like everything in this human world, is not for everybody. Some people find it difficult and inconvenient to follow this eating pattern while for some, the risks outweigh the benefits. Certain medical conditions are counter-indicative for intermittent fasting, and for such people, this eating pattern could be dangerous.

The set of people for whom intermittent fasting works perfectly are:

- Those with a history of maintaining and monitoring calorie intake.

- Those who follow a fixed physical exercise regimen.

- Those who are not bound by any kind of family problems including taking care of the elderly and children.

- Those who have supportive partners and indulge in this eating pattern together as a couple.

- Those who are in jobs in which you can lie low for short periods of time when you are adjusting into a new pattern.

Being male and having the considerations listed above give you an added advantage in making a great success of intermittent fasting. Being female has a few problems with intermittent fasting which is discussed later in this chapter.

The set of people for whom intermittent fasting works moderately well (with some adjustments and extra caution) are:

- Those who married and have children and elders to take care of.

- Those who have to interact with clients and are in stressed-out high-pressure jobs.

- Those who are in sports.

The first two require adjustments, most of which are doable with a bit of commitment and hard work. Here again, women who have the same problems as above tend to find it harder to achieve intermittent fasting goals compared to men.

Who Should Not Try It?

The set of people who should NOT attempt intermittent fasting include:

- Pregnant women.

- Those who have a history of bad eating habits.

- Those who are in a chronically-stressed out jobs.

- Those who have a problem sleeping.

- Those who are new to dieting and exercising.

If you are new to the concept of dieting and exercising, jumping into intermittent fasting is not a great idea. Get your basics right, get your eating disorders sorted out, take care of any nutritional deficiencies you have, and only then try intermittent fasting. Pregnant women need extra energy and so intermittent fasting is simply NOT for them. Also, if you are planning on starting a family, the women partners must not attempt intermittent fasting (more on this later in the chapter).

If you are under chronic stress and not sleeping well, then you too must NOT attempt intermittent fasting because you need to reduce stress to lead a normal life, and not add stress by skipping meals. Similarly, if you have a pattern of bad eating habits, then intermittent fasting will make your eating habits worse. Therefore, get your habits regulated before trying IF.

Other Reasons and Situations to Exercise Caution

Additionally, people with the following problems must not try intermittent fasting:

Food Sensitivities

Despite making the best plans in prepping and preparing meals, issues of food sensitivities will creep into your system with intermittent fasting. It is best to avoid this method if you are sensitive to any kind of food including gluten, soy, dairy, etc.

There are studies which reveal that intermittent fasting can trigger gut and brain problems that are connected to food sensitivities. These triggers from intermittent fasting can potentially create multiple health issues including leaky gut, inflammation, weight loss resistance, and more.

Moreover, intermittent fasting does not give you the liberty to eat what you want, right? These food sensitivities could create roadblocks in your meal-planning and leave very little in terms of nutritional sources. Therefore, it is best to avoid intermittent fasting if you have food sensitivities and allergies.

Stomach problems

If you have a history of stomach problems such as bloating, gas, and other post-meal issues, then intermittent fasting is not for you. While these stomach problems are temporary during the initial stages of intermittent fasting, if they persist or if you have a history of them, then you must not consider this eating pattern.

Again, restricted food intake can exacerbate gut issues because you are already restricting a lot of ingredients in your meals and increasing the stress to your system is not good for you. For example, sugars and even fruits juices typically are not allowed for people with gut issues. Now, while on an intermittent fast, if unwittingly or otherwise, you drink orange juice during your eating window and you have a history of gut problems, then you are going to get worse.

Anxiety and stress

If your life is already on an overdose of anxiety and stress, then intermittent fasting is only going to add to it. Therefore, it is not a great idea. In fact, the stress of not eating can be a simple trigger that brings forth anxieties from other aspects of your life. Studies have shown that stress hormones are increased during hunger.

Sleep issues

If you have a history of sleep issues, then avoid intermittent fasting. When you start off your regimen and find that you have problems going to sleep, then check for the kind of food you consume during dinner. Avoid high-carbs that result in a sugar rush making it difficult for you to fall asleep.

However, if after adjusting your meals correctly, you still

have a problem with sleep, then it might be a good idea to stop intermittent fasting, and speak to your physician first.

Adrenal fatigue

Caused by a malfunctioning or reduced efficiency of the adrenal glands; walnut-sized organs sitting atop your kidneys. They produce over 50 different types of hormones vital for efficient and healthy functioning body system. Two of the most important hormones produces by the adrenal glands are cortisol and dehydroepiandrosterone (DHEA).

Cortisol is directly connected to metabolism, stress response, blood-sugar control, and inflammation. DHEA is associated with estrogen and testosterone production. Fasting when the adrenal glands functions are compromised can cause more harm than good. Adrenal dysfunction is the time to reduce stresses of all kinds on your body, and to nourish it well; both of which cannot be achieved with intermittent fasting, at least during the initial adjustment periods.

Therefore, if your adrenal glands are not functioning at optimal levels, then intermittent fasting may not be the best option for you.

Low thyroid function

Another condition wherein you must exercise caution before starting off on an intermittent fasting eating pattern. A lot of people with compromised thyroid functions tend to gain weight quickly, and such people are easily tempted into taking the highly effective intermittent fasting path to weight loss.

However, you must exercise extreme caution, and should definitely speak to your physician before attempting it. Moreover, even if you do after your physician gives his or her approval, you must track your thyroid regularly to monitor and manage negative impacts from the added stress of intermittent fasting.

Intermittent Fasting and Women

At home, you might have noticed the differences in the eating pattern of your parents. Medical conditions aside, it is quite likely that your dad needed just one or two meals a day and rarely would want to eat first thing in the morning. Your mom, on the other hand, would get down to eating breakfast almost immediately on waking up and would eat 4-5 meals a day.

Yes, it is possible that both your parents are healthy and fine because their intake is managed in different but healthy ways. Women do tend to have more problems with intermittent fasting than men. While some women find it very easy to stick to their fasting schedules, many others have complained of multiple health issues.

Fasting and Hormones

Studies have proven that hormones connected to the reproductive system of women are extremely sensitive to energy and food intake. Here, for better understanding, I would have to explain certain hormones and how they affect the reproductive system.

The hypothalamic-pituitary-gonadal or the HPG axis represents the coordinating efforts of three critical endocrine glands. This HPG axis' job is to control hormonal traffic in your body. Here are the processes that take place:

- The hypothalamus first releases gonadotropin-releasing hormone or GnRH.

- The release of GnRH signals the pituitary gland to release a follicular stimulating hormone or FHS and luteinizing hormone or LH.

- FSH and LH now act on the testes and ovaries as follows:

  o In women, these two hormones trigger the production and release of progesterone and estrogen both of which are needed for ovulation and pregnancy.

o   In men, FSH and LH triggers sperm and testosterone production and release.

These processes and hormonal reactions and triggers need to be timed precisely to meet the regular, specific monthly cycle. When the timing goes haywire, the entire reproductive cycle could take a big hit. GnRH appears to be very sensitive to all environmental factors including fasting, and the processes get thrown off gear.

Studies have shown that even short-term fasting can bring about extreme changes in the hormonal functions of some women. There are studies which reveal that skipping a single meal alerts the body system and reacts very quickly to changes in energy consumption for some women. This could be the reason why IF works for some women and does not work for others.

While the reason for intermittent fasting to have a more significant effect on women's hormonal system than men's is still under investigation, some studies are connecting it to the functioning of protein-like molecules called kisspeptins. Neurons use kisspeptins to improve the efficacy of interaction among themselves resulting in increased productivity and sensitivity of the nervous system.

Kisspeptins, which are very sensitive to hunger and satiety hormones such as ghrelin, leptin, and insulin stimulates production and release of GnRH in both men and women. It is noticed that female mammals have an increased presence of kisspeptin as compared to males. Therefore, women are believed to be more sensitive to any changes to the energy balance in their bodies.

Based on these observations and theories, some experts believe that fasting brings about a drop in kisspeptin levels which, in turn, affects the other hormonal cycles making it more difficult for women to get desired results than men.

Fasting experiments done on rats have shown that the entire reproductive cycle went awry. Not only did kisspeptin levels become very low but also estradiol, a hormone that inhibits GnRH production, increased significantly. These experiments showed that it took about 10-15 days of fasting for the reproductive system to be disrupted.

While these experiments were only conducted on animals, similar results can be expected for humans too, considering the deep connection between the functioning of reproductive hormones, appetite, and energy balance in the body.

While missing a few periods might appear to be a harmless side-effect of fasting especially if you are not looking to have kids in the near future, you must remember that metabolism and the female reproductive system are deeply connected. Hormonal imbalances can affect even those aspects that are not related to getting pregnant.

Here is an illustration of an example of a potential effect of fasting on some women. Typically, women eat a lesser amount of proteins than men. During fasting, this amount is further reduced. Amino acids, the nutrient from proteins, are essential for multiple metabolic activities.

For example, amino acids are responsible for activating estrogen receptors. They are also needed for the synthesis of insulin-like growth factor (IGF-1) which triggers the thickening of the uterine walls to set the ball rolling for the reproductive cycle. Therefore, low-protein diets can potentially affect fertility and libido.

Moreover, estrogen is a hormone that is used in functions other than reproduction too. Estrogen receptors are found all over our body including bones, the digestive system, and our brain. If the estrogen balance is affected, a variety of metabolic functions including moods, cognitive ability, digestion, recovery, bone formation, and more get affected.

Estrogen plays an important role in energy balance and appetite too. They trigger the full and hungry feelings by modifying peptides such as ghrelin (for hunger) and cholecystokinin (for feeling full). Estrogens stimulate those neurons in the hypothalamus responsible for the production and release of appetite-regulating peptides.

Therefore, some women tend to overeat when there is a drop in their estrogen levels. Fasting can potentially create such problems. Estrogens are critical metabolic regulators.

The effect of estrogens does not stop here. There are three different estrogen metabolites including estrone, estriol, and estradiol. The ratios of these three metabolites, whose exact roles are still being studied, are continually changing.

However, it is seen that estradiol levels are high before menopause, and drops after menopause. Some experts opine that this drop in estradiol levels could increase fat storage in some women; the connection being fat is needed for the production of estradiol. This explanation could be the reason why some women find it difficult to lose fat after menopause.

Considering the importance of estrogen and other female hormones, it makes sense to take care of your reproductive health instead of trying intermittent fasting, especially if your body is sensitive. Interestingly, there are many women for whom intermittent fasting works fine. So, it is up to you to investigate how things work for you and then take a cautious approach. It might make sense not to endeavor intermittent fasting if you are trying to get pregnant. Whatever the case, speak to your physician and make an informed decision.

Common and Avoidable Intermittent Fasting Mistakes

Despite what has been said in this chapter regarding people for whom intermittent fasting is not a good idea, there is little doubt that for most of us this eating pattern can work very well, helping us gain lean mass while dropping body fat. Even for people like us, things can go wrong if we don't take about certain elements such as setting unrealistic expectations. If you can take care to avoid falling into common pitfalls that most novices tend to get trapped by, there is no reason why IF cannot be an effective means of losing weight and achieving healthy living. Here are some of the top common mistakes you must, and with a bit of care, can avoid:

Eating Junk Food in Your Eating Window

A common complaint from many novices is they are unable to lose weight or fat despite 'strictly' following the 16:8 or 18:6 or any other IF method. If you were to look at what these people were eating in your eating window, you would be able to find the mistake easily.

You must remember that nothing can prevent your

downward slide from a healthy life if you don't stop eating junk food. Eating wholesome and nutritious food in your eating window while you are on an intermittent fasting phase is imperative for effective fat and weight loss.

So, if you are not losing weight as expected, re-evaluate and re-plan your meals to include only wholesome food. Refer to Chapter 8 to know what can be eaten and what should be avoided in your meals.

Not being active during the fasting window

Idle hands during your fasting window can be counterproductive. Avoid doing nothing during that time. Schedule your usual activity as if you are not fasting. It might make sense, however, to avoid intense training and exercise schedules.

When your body and mind are busy on an important activity, psychological hunger will not affect you. You will be too focused on your work to be distracted by hunger pangs and cravings. Also, avoid hanging out with people who are constantly on an eating spree. Don't visit the canteen or break room during the coffee break. You could bring your own herbal teas and drink it at your desk.

The fasting period is actually great to give vent to your creativity because more of the body energy is available to improve brain functioning, repair, and rejuvenation. After the initial days of a bit of slack, you will notice your energy levels are better during the fasting period than during the eating period. So, avoid leading a dull, activity-less life during your fasting period, and just do everything normally.

Don't Overdo on Stimulants

It is common for intermittent fasters to start the day with coffee and skip breakfast. And typically, 2-3 cups of coffee or tea are downed before the first meal of the day later on. If you don't watch out, it is possible to convert your morning time into a caffeinated period where you are downing cups and cups of coffee.

A couple of coffees are fine because they help you manage hunger pangs. However, getting addicted to caffeine so much that it becomes a meal itself is a bad idea. Get your coffee fix, that's ok. Just remember not to overdo it.

Unrealistic Expectations

Reaching the 18:6 fasting daily or the Once-a-Day Warrior Diet might be your ultimate goal. However, expecting to do that from Day 1 is not just naïve but also detrimental to your health. Firstly, starting off on an intense fast without giving your body sufficient time to get used to the new eating regimen could trigger unpleasant effects including drastic changes in your metabolism. Second, setting unrealistic goals is one of the primary reasons for not being able to meet your IF goals.

In the initial days, avoid setting ambitious goals and being too hard on yourself. Moving from 4-5 meals to wholesome foods once or twice a day is an extreme step that is bound to fail. Instead, start gradually, and slowly increase your intensity. See Chapter 7 for a flexible and straightforward plan to kick-start your intermittent fasting.

Being Afraid of Hunger

Fear of hunger is a huge thing for many intermittent fasting novices. Hunger is a natural and perfectly tolerable aspect of human life. Fasting for 16-18 hours a day will neither result in death nor will your muscles waste away. Only your digestive system will be given some much-needed rest from overworking. Manage hunger pangs and cravings sensibly using the tips and tricks provided in Chapter 5.

Thinking More is Always Better

If you have had success with intermittent fasting with the 16:8 method, and you think you will lose more weight and fat if you extended your fasting time to 18-20 hours, you could be right or wrong. You need not be always right in thinking that extending your fasting period for longer durations will give you better results. If you are fasting more than 20 hours a day, and still not losing weight, then you should re-evaluate your choices, and make some changes other than extending your fasting period.

Getting Obsessed about Time

Obsessing about the time of eating and fasting can be a big stress element for you. The happiest benefit of intermittent fasting is the flexibility it offers in terms of when to eat and, more or less, what to eat also. In your eating window, eat when you are hungry. Don't think that if you don't eat, then you'll have problems later on.

If hunger has not set in yet, munch a few raw vegetables. If your dinner time comes at 6 pm on a day instead of 8 pm, don't panic. Eat if you are hungry. Else, find another alternative that is suitable for you on that day. Don't allow the clock to run your life when you choose the IF way.

Not Being Patient

Many people start fasting and are so impatient to lose weight that they spend the entire time not eating, and then overeating because they do not have the patience to listen to their body and heed its warnings. Such people treat intermittent fasting as a magic trick, and when results don't happen magically, they think it is not a great way to lose weight, and go back to their old ways.

Understand it takes time, effort, and energy for effective results to happen with intermittent fasting. It is not a magic pill. Being impatient for results will have unfavorable outcomes for you.

Unfortunately, impatience also breeds another mistake, and that is to give up too soon. The lack of unrealistic expectations driven by impatience makes some people become undisciplined leading to worse energy and weight situations than before. If you keep jumping off from the bandwagon, your body is going to get confused, and it is going to find different ways to rebel, increasing your discomfort and unpleasantness.

Therefore, you must wait out the difficult phase with patience and give your body and mind time to get accustomed to the new pattern, and sooner than later, you will see great results. But, you have to be patient with yourself.

Thinking the Sum of the Parts Always Add Up

People who think like this obsess over little things like, 'Should it be 18:6 or 17.5:6.5?' or 'I've put a teaspoon of

cream in my coffee today, will it ruin my entire plan?'
You can try to understand each piece separately, and yet,
sometimes that little piece works differently when put
together with other pieces.

If you start eating a few minutes before your designated
eating window, it is perfectly fine. Alternately, don't
think you have to eat the last bite at the precise last
second of your eating window. Avoid obsessing over
each little piece because there are layers in the entire
exercise which are not just beyond your control, but you
are not even aware of some of them. Instead, focus on
pertinent elements of your intermitting fasting plan like:

- Is my food selection right?

- Am I engaged in sufficient physical activity?

- Am I getting adequate amounts of macro- and
  micronutrients?

- Am I eating enough fruit and vegetables?

Focus on the large issues, and resolve challenges as and
when you encounter them. Here are some important
elements that truly add up to the sum of the parts: Your
day should be divided into eating and fasting periods
with the fasting period being at least 12 hours. Slowly
work towards making the eating period as small as
possible. Make sure your meals are primarily wholesome
and nutritious. Don't be obsessed with mistakes you

make wittingly or unwittingly with your food intake occasionally. Pick up the thread from where you stopped and move on.

Take a cautious, gradual approach to this science-approved and ancient method of intermittent fasting, and persist with your efforts before expecting tangible results. Don't force your body into the intermittent fasting method. While it is true that our ancestors lived like this, and were far healthier than we are today, some of our bodies are simply not made for intermittent fasting.

If you have tried hard enough, and have taken care of all possible loopholes, and been persistent in your efforts, and still do not see any improvement, it is perfectly in order to re-evaluate if intermittent fasting is the right method for you or not. If you think intermittent fasting is a constant struggle and a daily battle that is draining your physical, mental, and emotional energy, feel free to try something else.

Chapter 7

7-Day Kick-Start

Intermittent Fasting Plan

Now, that you know a lot about intermittent fasting including its umpteen benefits, and you want to give it a shot, where should you begin? You already know that fasting is not the same as starving, and therefore, you do not need to conjure up images of suffering and starvation.

It is so easy to fall for this seemingly 'horror' image of waking up in the morning and starting the timer for the next meal which is not immediate. People begin to imagine how they will feel when they eat their first bite after the period of fasting, and the anxiety of the wait only increases. It doesn't have to be this bad at all.

Before you jump into your regimen, here are some tips and suggestions to make your fasting journey a success.

Indicators of a Successful Fasting Regimen

While fasting might appear to be merely giving up food for a predetermined period of time, other factors count towards the success of a fasting regimen.

- Your objectives and goals from the fasting regimen are clear. You know exactly what you want from your intermittent fasting approach.

- You can easily complete the fasting period you have set for yourself with relative ease. For example, avoid setting fasting periods that are beyond your capability. There is no point in setting a 21-day period fast, then eating on the fifth day because you felt like it, and continuing the fast on the 6th day. Therefore, keep your fasting periods realistic and doable.

- Healing benefits are optimized during the fasting window. Excessive physical activity should be avoided during this time.

- Exercising (to lose more weight) during the fasting window typically should not be done at all because it can be counterproductive to your initial goals. Moreover, intense exercising during the fasting window is contrary to the true nature of fasting.

- You can easily move in and out of your fasting windows with little or no health issues.

- You eat wholesome, healthy, and nutritious meals during the eating window, and continuously work to improve your lifestyle quality.

- You can keep off the weight you have lost at the end of the fasting period.

If you can achieve the indicators mentioned above, then your fasting regimen is a big success. Fasting is not a one-time diet fad. It is a holistic attitude to change your mental, emotional, spiritual, and physical approach to a fit and healthy life. Avoid using fasting as a method to fix your bad dietary habits and emotional eating disorders. If you do so, intermittent fasting can have a negative impact on your health and overall lifestyle.

Tips To Achieve Intermittent Fasting Success

Before embarking on your intermittent fasting journey, you must prepare yourself to achieve success. Here are some tips for the preparation process:

Identify the goals of fasting

Clear fasting goals are your foundation and anchor throughout your fasting journey. If you don't have clear-set goals, you will find it difficult to stick to your fasting plan. Work out the reasons why you want to fast. Make detailed entries in your fasting journal. In fact, your goals should be the first page of your fasting journal. For example, I want to fast to achieve an improved approach to eating. Or I want to fast to lose x kg of weight.

Keeping these goals handy and in the first page of your fasting journal will help you feel a connection to your fasting journey and will drive commitment. Answer the following questions as part of your goal-setting mechanism:

- Why do you want to fast?

- What do you want to achieve by fasting?

Detailed answers to these questions will help you stay on course. The clearer your goals are, the easier it will be to achieve them through fasting.

Get the right frame of mind

Get into fasting only when your mind is fully prepared and ready for it. Once your mind is ready to accept and face the challenges, your body will find it very easy to follow suit. Get into the fasting regimen with full intention to achieve your goals. Here are some tips:

- Read up plenty of information about fasting. Bookmark your favorite pages so that you can access them whenever you need to.

- Read up on other people's fasting journals.

- Eat your favorite and most indulgent food for the last time and promise yourself that the next time you eat this will be only after you have achieved your fasting goals.

All these deliberate preparation mechanisms will put your mind in the right frame to begin fasting thereby enhancing the chance of achieving success without excessive cravings and desires. Hesitation before even starting off is going to deter your chances of success. Prepare your body and mind, and dive in with full intent. The deeper your intent, the higher the chances of success!

Avoid creating a panic situation in your mind

Prepping your mind into the right frame is good. Panicking is bad. There is no way any major damage is going to happen if you decide to take the intermittent fasting way. You are not getting into some long-drawn fasting mechanism of more than a day which will never result in any bad consequences.

The worst side-effect of even a 24-hour fast is only the gnawing effects of hunger pangs. Other than that, just tell yourself that your next meal is just a few hours away. Therefore, stop creating a panic situation and simply enjoy the process of getting healthier and giving your body the freedom from having to work on its digestion constantly.

Avoid talking about your intermittent fasting regimen with others

Other than having to take a clearance from your physician if you have a history of medical illness, there is no need to talk to anybody about your decision to try intermittent fasting.

In addition to hunger pangs and other initial challenges, you will also have to deal with unnecessary reactions from others. If you have family and friends who are open to alternate lifestyle therapies, then they could be supportive of your methods. However, those who are not open to new ideas will not be supportive and could react negatively to your approach. It's better to do so without such negativity.

Remember intermittent fasting is not some fad diet or quick fix

Intermittent fasting can help you lose weight and have a healthier lifestyle than before. It can help you see through your food weaknesses and help you overcome them. It can create an amazing balance in your physical, emotional, and mental state. However, all this is possible only if you follow through with diligence and patience.

You must recognize intermittent fasting as a form of healing that will last a lifetime and not some quick fix that needs to be done for a short while after which you can get back to your old lifestyle. It is a slow, healthy, and sustainable way to reset bad eating habits, detox mentally and physically, and lead a more fulfilling life than before. It is NOT a quick fix.

Be ready to manage your emotions while you fast

Along with food cravings, you are bound to deal with a lot of negative emotions that will surface as you change your eating pattern. Skipping meals will free your body and mind and find ways to clear up elements you have brushed under the carpet because you have not had the resources (primarily, time and energy) to deal with them. Be ready for these emotions and work through them. Here are a few tips:

- First, identify the emotions. It is quite likely that you get hit with a variety of emotions all at once. Recognize as many of them as you can, and then choose one (invariably anger is the most evident one) to work with. You can move on to the others when you have handled the first one.

- Second, delve deep and find answers for this emotion. Initially, you will get answers such as, 'my life is unfair,' or 'everybody else is having fun,' or something general statements like this. Persist and probe deeper, and you will find real answers staring back at you, many of them the past unmanaged events in your life.

- Once you have recognized the event(s) that create the anger, find out how exactly those events led to this emotion. Remember that events are all objective, and only when you attach emotions to the events, they become subjective interpretations of the situation. These emotions are quite independent of the event or situation.

- When you look at the emotions, connect them to the actual events in your life, you will find the necessary closure.

- Move on to the next emotion and repeat the above steps.

124

The emotional detox that happens when you indulge in intermittent fasting is a result of all these emotional closures!

Remember to get ready to break your fast correctly

Getting this right is an extremely critical element for success. There is no point in fasting if you choose to sit with a tub of ice-cream and burgers to break your fast. In fact, most people are under the wrong impression that getting into the fasting window is more difficult than breaking the fast to get into the eating window. Nothing can be farther from the truth. Easing yourself in a healthy manner into the eating window is a bigger challenge.

Fasting windows put your digestive system into a short slumber and dumping high-calorie food immediately after breaking your fast can be dangerous. The longer your fasting period is, the more care you need to give to the kind of food you eat when you break your fast.

7-Day Kick-Start Intermittent Fasting Plan

Keeping the pre-fasting tips in mind, here is a 7-day kick-start intermittent fasting plan that is very likely to succeed for beginners. This plan is a daily intermittent plan that gradually extends your fasting period by 2 hours at each stage. By the end of the week, you will be one day into the 18:6 method of intermittent fasting, which is the ideal place to be in for maximum fat loss and health gain.

Day 1 and 2

On these two days, continue your earlier practice of eating 4 meals a day starting with breakfast after 8 hours of sleep and finishing your dinner at 8 pm the previous night. Typically, most of us have this 10-hour fasting mechanism already built into our body system. So, simply continue this for the first two days.

However, focus on regulating your eating time more precisely than before. Focus on eliminating snacks completely from your eating pattern. Calculate your calorie needs and work towards keeping your calorie intake slightly less than your daily needs. Be conscious of what you eat and when you eat. Get your food and fasting journal ready.

Make sure your meals are planned and prepped so that only wholesome, nutritious foods are consumed. Get mentally prepared during these two days to start intermittent fasting. Giving up snacking will be the biggest challenge here. Make entries diligently in your journal.

Day 3 and 4

With the tips to prepare your body and mind before jumping into intermittent fasting, and the first two days dedicated to preparing physically by cutting down snacks and unwholesome food, your body will be quite ready to skip breakfast. Skipping breakfast is an excellent jump-off point for beginners of intermittent fasting.

By skipping the first meal of your day, you are moving your fasting period from 10 hours (including 8 hours) spent sleeping to 12 hours, and eating an early brunch at around 10 am. The most challenging part of skipping breakfast is in the mind because nearly all of us have been conditioned into thinking that breakfast is the most important meal of the day that shouldn't be missed.

Why is breakfast not the most important meal of the day? – There are multiple studies which have proven that eating breakfast has no significant effect on your weight loss program. People who ate and those who didn't eat breakfast lost similar amounts of weight with all other elements such as exercise and calorie consumption remaining the same.

The biggest problem with 'breakfast-is-the-most-important-meal-of-the-day' is that your meal plans get very restricted. If you are a person who does not like to skip eating, and you are compelled to eat breakfast because of myths created around the meal, you are bound to eat more than you need. It restricts your ability to plan your meals to suit your needs and your lifestyle.

Irrespective of what research says, it is important for you to find what ticks for you and choose that. In this plan, if you are more of a breakfast person, then make sure you skip dinner so that your fasting period gets extended from 8 hours to 12 hours.

Why is the timing of your meals not important too? – The timing of your meals doesn't really matter. If you have to eat 1500 calories a day, you can choose to have 4 meals of 375 calories each or 5 meals of 300 calories each; it's all the same to your body. The composition of your meals does matter, of course. Intermittent fasting entails you to skip one of the 375-calorie or 300-calorie meals so that you reduce your overall daily calorie intake.

Don't allow psychological dependence on timing your meals to get your intermittent fasting right. Skip breakfast and move seamlessly into the 12-hour fasting regimen.

Once you have mastered these two days, and have learned to disregard the myth surrounding breakfast, then you can easily get into the 12-hour fasting regimen by simply starting off your day with a cup of coffee. In addition, you will get more free time to do other things.

Nearly 90% of the people in an intermittent fasting regimen skip breakfast. Very few people such as those who have strenuous training regimens in the morning or those who simply prefer skipping lunch or dinner instead don't skip breakfast.

It takes very little time to adjust to this new routine of skipping breakfast, and you can move into the next stage very easily.

Day 5 and 6

In this stage, move your lunch to 12 pm giving you a 16 hour fasting period from the previous dinner time of 8 pm. Each time, you are extending your fasting period by two hours only. Your body and mind will easily adjust to this gradual process, and fit in well. By this stage, you are spending more time fasting than eating. At this level, you can fit in 3 meals between 12 noon and 8 pm.

Day 7

However, the ideal intermittent fasting is an 18-hour fasting period wherein you eat 2 meals between 2 pm and 8 pm which is the next stage, to be tried only on Day 7 after your body has got adjusted the 16 hours of fasting. This is the most difficult stage of intermittent fasting. However, it is that stage that burns the most amount of fat and at the optimum rate without tiring you out unnecessarily because you are consuming two nutritious, wholesome meals on a daily basis.

You Can Do Your Own Thing

There are no hard and fast rules to follow the 7-day regimen mentioned above. You can make any of the following changes you think is better suited for your needs and lifestyle:

- You don't have to start at Stage 1 (Day 1 and 2) if you have tried intermittent fasting on and off earlier before. It means you can directly jump into the Day 3 and 4 stage by shelving your breakfast by 2 hours.

- You can remain at each stage for as long as you are losing weight. However, the two-day gap for each stage will give your body sufficient motivation to take on the next stage without excessive issues. If you stayed very long at one stage, it is possible that moving to the next stage could prove difficult, and you would have to break the hunger pang cycle again with difficulty. Remember, you need to get to the 16:8 or 18:6 stage for effective intermittent fasting benefits to set in.

- Nothing can stop you from diving straight into the 16:8 regimen. However, is your body ready for this huge jump? There is no value in fixing unrealistic fasting durations that you cannot live up. Breaking fasts before time will not give you benefits, and also will leave unhappy and dissatisfied with the entire exercise. Take things slowly, and work at a pace that you are comfortable with.

- Use tips from Chapter 4 on dealing with hunger pangs.

- The important thing is to keep moving forward. Don't allow yourself to fall more than one level. So, if you are at the Day 5 and 6 level, then do everything in your power to not fall to the Day 1 and 2 level. It gets more difficult to climb back two rungs of the ladder. It is not such a big challenge to climb back one rung.

More Tips for Beginners

There is no universally right way to achieving success in your intermittent fasting journey. The most effective way of increasing the chances of success is by gathering as much information and knowledge you can before you plunge in. Additionally, as you progress, you are bound to encounter expected and unexpected challenges, all of which need to be overcome if you want to reach the end of the road. Here are more tips to help you on the way:

Choose A Plan That Is Aligned With Your Lifestyle And Suits Your Needs

The types of intermittent fasting have already been discussed in Chapter 2. Reread it, and find which method suits you best. The most effective way is the one that is explained in this chapter in the previous section; to start slowly and increase the fasting duration by two hours at each stage.

However, if you find that you are able to do it faster or you need to slow down the pace, feel free to do so. The important thing is to be comfortable and at ease, especially during the initial stages when your body is getting accustomed to the changes.

For example, although the above plan is to start with skipping breakfast, if it is easier for you to skip dinner because your bedtime is earlier (again, because your day starts as early as 5 am), then that works out too. Just remember to increase the fasting period in batches, and give your body time to adjust to the new regimen.

Take Baby Steps

Even if you are very confident about your body's metabolic activity, and know exactly how it behaves, as a beginner to intermittent fasting, it is critical that you take baby steps initially. It would be foolhardy to jump into the 16:8 method on Day 1. Take baby steps for

132

sustainable results.

Hydration Is Essential

Perhaps, I have repeated this element earlier too in the book. However, I will not hesitate to add it as a special point in this section. As a beginner, you have to remember that hydrating your body during the fasting period is essential for success, and to prevent other health issues. Black tea and coffee and sparkling water are the best options for hydration.

Let Your Meals Be Wholesome and Sufficient

One of the benefits of intermittent fasting is that you don't have to scrimp on calories during the eating window. Yes, the quality of calories does matter. However, don't stop with a measly salad and call it a meal. Ensure you eat foods that include all macronutrients in all the meals. Feel free to include your favorite cookie or that small ounce of pasta. Just remember to keep an overall track of your calorie intake so that you are in a calorie deficit state.

Don't Binge-Eat During Your Eating Window

Yes, you don't need to scrimp on calories; but, you cannot overdo it too. Don't binge during your eating window. A great tip to avoid bingeing, especially during the first meal after your fasting period, is to eat a handful of nuts and small bowl fruits first. This approach will take the edge off your hunger. Wait for about 30-60 minutes before you eat your big meal. You will eat more sensibly.

Avoid Excessive Workouts During The Fasting Window

At the beginning of your intermittent fasting, it might make sense to stop going to the gym. Give your body time to adjust to a completely new and strange eating pattern. Don't add the stress of excessive workouts to it. Instead, take a brisk walk or indulge in yoga or tai chi to stay active and conserve calories.

Once you get accustomed to IF, then you can restart your gym membership. Even now, it might be a good idea to choose a time that coincides with your eating window rather than your fasting window. Listen to what your body is saying, and follow the signs diligently.

Keep Track Of Your Progress

Tangible results are great motivators to stay on track. Don't forget to track your progress using the methods explained in Chapter 5.

Chapter 8

What and When to Eat

The importance of eating right during the eating window cannot be undermined. Eating the wrong kinds and wrong quantities of food will defeat the very purpose of intermittent fasting. While there is really no restriction on what foods to eat during the eating window, a huge Mac-and-Cheese with fries on the side will not help you achieve your intermittent fasting goals of losing weight and healthy living.

A well-balanced meal that combines all nutrients is essential for effective results from intermittent fasting. You must focus on consuming nutrient-rich foods such as fruit and vegetables, nuts and seeds, whole grains, dairy products, and lean proteins. All your meals should essentially be made with unprocessed, whole-grain, and fresh ingredients.

Also, you must include a bit of variety in your meals in terms of flavor and texture which will reduce feelings of hunger during your fasting period. Here are some elements that can be great inclusions in your diet while you are on an intermittent fasting regimen.

What to Eat and Drink During Your Eating Window

Water - The importance of hydration has been discussed in different sections of Chapter 4. Water is the basic element that keeps every organ in your body healthy and working efficiently. The amount of water needed to be consumed varies from person to person. A good method to check if you are drinking sufficient quantities of water is to see that the color of your urine pale yellow. Dark yellow urine is the first indicator of dehydration. Effects of dehydration include headaches, giddiness, and fatigue.

Lack of water coupled with limited intake of food is nothing but a recipe for disaster. There are sound, scientific reasons to limit the intake of food. But, there is no need to limit zero-calorie water, an essential element for all body metabolisms. If you are bored with plain water, add a dash of lime with a sprig of mint, to freshen up your glass. Here are some more tips to make plain water taste lovely:

Add fresh fruit juices – You can add a dash of lime, lemon, or orange zest to flavor your plain water. You could also add cucumber slices or strawberries/watermelon crushes. A sprig of mint will go well with all these flavors. Be wary of some fruit juices that could stimulate your taste buds which, in turn, could increase hunger pangs.

Drink a bubbly – Drinking sparkling mineral water instead of plain water will taste better as well as increase the intake of essential minerals into your body. You can carbonate your water and makes a seltzer. Add natural juice flavors to enhance the taste.

Drink tea – There are varieties of zero-calories teas available in the market including red, green, white, fruit, and herbal teas. With negligible amounts of caffeine and a wide variety of flavors to choose from, tea can be a delicious replacement for plain water during your fasting window.

Avocados – Filled with fabulous fats, avocados perform the magic trick of keeping you satiated and full for long hours. Include avocados in at least one meal of the day. There are studies which have proven that people who ate avocados did not suffer from hunger pangs for much longer periods than those who did not consume these creamy-textured fruits. Here are more benefits of including avocados in your meal that could combat challenges faced during intermittent fasting:

Nutrient-dense fruit - The loss of nutrients is one of the primary concerns for people on intermittent fasting. Avocados can be the answer for such people. The wonder fruit is a rich source of Vitamin K, Folate, Potassium, Vitamin C, Vitamin B5, Vitamin B6, and Vitamin E. Eating one avocado will take care of all the essential micronutrients your body needs for healthy living.

Contains monosaturated fatty acids – The majority of this fat-rich food is oleic acid, a mono-saturated fatty acid that promotes heart health.

Fiber-rich – The indigestible matter of avocados (the fiber in it) is excellent for weight loss. You don't have to worry about another ingredient to get your fibers. Moreover, avocados are rich in both soluble and insoluble fibers. While soluble fibers are important for gut flora, the insoluble fibers are great for improved bowel movements, both of which are excellent for weight loss.

Delicious and can be easily integrated into your meals – Make a salad, add them to various recipes, or simply scoop out the fruit and eat it straight away. This delicious wonder fruit can be easily integrated into your meals.

Fish – Fish is a rich source of proteins and healthy fats. It contains a lot of Vitamin D as well. Considering your nutrient intake is going to be limited while on the intermittent fasting regimen, it is best to include nutrient-rich and tasty fish into your dishes. Moreover, fish is believed to improve cognitive benefits too. After all, it is referred to by experts and believers as the 'brain food.'

Vegetables from the cabbage family – Referred to as cruciferous vegetables, these include Brussels sprouts, broccoli, and cauliflower. Rich in fibers, these veggies are great especially during intermittent fasting when eating patterns are a bit erratic. The fiber-rich cruciferous veggies will help manage constipation, a temporary setback that most beginners face. Fiber also helps you by making you feel full for a longer period of time thereby helping you manage hunger during the fasting window.

Potatoes – Yes, you heard right. Potatoes are great for intermittent fasters as they are rich in good carbohydrates. Studies have proven that this vegetable is one of the most satiating ingredients available to man. Of course, chips and French fries should NOT be treated as potatoes. Here are some healthy ways of cooking potatoes:

Baking – with its skin on is the healthiest way of cooking potatoes as this form of cooking minimizes loss of nutrients in the best possible way. You can bake it whole with the skin or cut into fingers, like French fries, and enjoy your fries, guilt-free.

Boiling with the skin on – Boiling any vegetables including potatoes can eliminate some essential nutrients such as water-soluble vitamins (vitamin C and B vitamins). Boiling potatoes along with skin minimizes loss of nutrients.

Ensure you stop cooking potatoes as soon as they become tender. Avoid overcooking potatoes. Also, boil in as little water as possible. Steaming is also a great idea to stem nutrient-loss. Don't throw away the excess water in which the vegetables were boiled. You can use it as vegetable stock for other recipes.

Another important thing to keep in mind while eating potatoes is your accompaniments. Don't add in huge amounts of butter, cream, cheese, or any kind of artificial flavoring. You are only enhancing the calories without any addition of food nutrients. Just drizzle some olive oil before baking. Use dried or fresh herbs as much as you want. Also, you can top baked potatoes with Greek yogurt or avocados.

Beans and Legumes – These low-carb and high-protein wonder ingredients are perfect for intermittent fasters, especially for the vegetarians who cannot sufficient proteins from fish and meat. Include chickpeas, lentils, and beans into your meals. They help to decrease body weight and have very little calories. Here are some of the healthiest beans that you must stock up in your kitchen cupboard before starting off on your intermittent fasting diet:

Chickpeas – A great source of folate and fibers, chickpeas are very low in calories. These beans are known to have multiple health benefits including reduction in blood sugar and blood cholesterol levels and improve gut health.

Lentils – Excellent sources of vegetable proteins, lentils can be amazing additions to soups and stews.

Peas – With a wide variety of peas to choose from, you can make every dish you make taste different. Again, a great source of protein and fiber, peas help in improving gut health.

Kidney beans – Often eaten together with rice, these are the most commonly used type of legumes across the world. In addition to its high fiber content, kidney beans are known to reduce blood sugar levels, a metabolic incident that usually occurs immediately after a meal.

Black beans – Excellent source of folate, fiber, and proteins, black beans also help in controlling the sudden blood-sugar spikes usually seen after a high-carb meal.

Soybeans – The source of delicious tofu, soybean is a favorite legume in Asia. A rich source of anti-oxidants, soybeans are known to reduce risks of multiple diseases including cancer and heart disorders. They also help in limiting loss of bone density during menopause.

Peanuts – Yes, peanuts are legumes and not nuts. They are rich in monosaturated fats and are believed to improve heart health.

Beans and legumes are an underestimated range of healthy ingredients. All of them are rich in dietary fiber, vegetable proteins, and other minerals and vitamins. Add them to your soups, stews, or any other recipes, and watch your food getting transformed into a nutritious and healthy meal.

Probiotics – Your gut is filled with extremely useful bacteria that are essential for efficient functioning of your digestive system. These bacteria in your gut need food consistently to do their job well. During intermittent fasting, when the gut is empty of food for a long period of time, the gut flora is bound to rebel and create discomfort for you in the form of constipation, a bloating feeling, etc.

You must include probiotic-rich foods to manage these discomforts. Excellent sources of probiotics include fermented foods such as tempeh, kimchi, kraut, kombucha, kefir, and soy products. You can also get readily available probiotic shots from the market. Here are more reasons for you to include probiotics in your meals, especially for intermittent fasters:

Balancing the gut flora and preventing discomforts – Probiotics are living organisms that help in restoring the balance of gut flora which, in turn, results in health benefits.

Treating and preventing diarrhea - Probiotics help to treat and prevent diarrhea, irrespective of how the problem cropped up.

Reducing symptoms of digestive disorders – During intermittent fasting, your digestive system is a little bit unbalanced, at least initially, which if ignored or untreated lead to potential gastrointestinal diseases such as IBS and ulcerative colitis. Probiotics are known to reduce the symptoms from these problems.

Berries – Smoothies made with berries are ideal as a first meal at the start of your eating window. Rich in vital nutrients including Vitamin C and flavonoids, berries are believed to even help in decreasing BMI when consumed over a long period of time. Include berries in your smoothies, salads, jams, and more and enjoy the taste, texture, and health benefits of amazing strawberries, blueberries, blackberries, and more.

Eggs – One large-sized egg contains 6 gm of proteins and is extremely easy to cook. Therefore, eggs are a brilliant addition to one of your meals. Getting sufficient quantities of proteins is essential for building and maintenance of muscle and overall health. Moreover, eating eggs creates a longer feeling of fullness as compared to many other foods.

Nuts – While nuts may contain a lot more calories than other snacks, the most critical difference is they are rich in 'good fat.' There are multiple studies which prove that the polyunsaturated fats in walnuts change the physiological markers associated with satiety and hunger. That means you don't get hit by hunger pangs for a long time during your fasting period if you ate some walnuts.

Whole Grains – Carbs are essential for intermittent fasters. However, the source of these carbs from the grains you use should be investigated. There are primarily three types of grains including whole grains, refined grains, and enriched grains.

Whole-grains – These are unmilled grains and retain their germ and bran which is removed by milling. All nutrients in whole-grains are intact. In addition to being a rich source of fiber, whole-grains contain plenty of critical nutrients including magnesium, selenium, and potassium. Whole-grains are available as single foods like popcorn kernels, brown rice, wheat, etc. and also as ingredients in various products such as whole wheat in whole-wheat bread, buckwheat in buckwheat pancakes, etc.

Refined grains – are milled and lose their bran and germ is removed in the milling process. Grains are milled and stripped off some of their essential nutrients including fiber to render a longer life and finer texture. Refined grains include white rice, white flour, de-germed corn flour, and foods made with these refined grains.

Enriched grains – In this type of grains, some of the nutrients lost during the milling process are added back it the grains later on. Nearly all refined grains are enriched, and some of the enriched grains are fortified with other minerals not found naturally in the food. So, fortified grains are enriched with iron and folic acid. Although enriched grains contain traces of important minerals, many of the naturally-found nutrients, especially fiber, are lost during processing.

Therefore, avoiding all other sources of carbs except

whole grains is your best choice. Whole-grain examples are brown rice, barley, bulgur wheat, millet, oatmeal, popcorn, pasta, bread, and crackers made with whole-wheat, and wild rice. Fiber- and protein-rich whole grains help in keeping you satiated for a long period of time. Here are some tips on how to include whole grains in your meals:

- Breakfast eaters can use whole-grain cereals like oatmeal, shredded wheat, and bran flakes.

- Replace plain white bread with whole-grain or whole-wheat bread and bagels.

- Replace pastries with low-fat bran muffins.

- Make your sandwiches with whole-grain rolls or wheat bread.

- Replace white-flour tortillas with whole-wheat options.

- White rice can be substituted with brown rice, bulgur, kasha, or wild rice.

- Use crushed bran cereal or rolled oats in place of bread crumbs in your recipes.

There are difficulties in choosing the right kind of whole-grain products. For example, if you choose brown bread thinking it is made of whole-wheat, think again because it could be a food color added to the bread. If in doubt, always read the label containing nutritional facts and ensure the product uses ONLY whole-grains and not a percentage amount.

What Not to Eat or Drink During Your Fasting Period

The concept of fasting is 'not eating.' So, ideally, you must NOT eat anything during your fasting period. Yet, staying hydrated during fasting is important and, therefore, you must be able to drink something without affecting the metabolism in your body. Here is that one ingredient you must NOT include in your hydrating drinks during the fasting period:

Sugar – Do NOT use any kinds of sugars or sugar substitutes in your hydrating drink. Tea with sugar, water with honey, etc. all has calories in them. Drinking sugared drinks is equivalent to breaking your fast and giving your body the glucose hit it is looking for to stop its fat metabolism.

In fact, there are studies which show that even zero-calorie sweeteners such as stevia, sucralose, and other artificial sweeteners spike blood-insulin levels taking your body off the fat metabolism path thereby defeating the very purpose of fasting. If you are very attached to your sweetened drinks, then include them in your eating window and account for the calories too.

Timing of Meals: Is It Better To Skip Breakfast or Dinner?

It is a common belief that it is better for fat loss if you eat earlier during the day rather than later at night. This approach has been in existence for a long time now and the clichéd proverb, "Eat breakfast like a king, lunch like a prince, and dinner like a pauper' is doing the rounds even today.

Now, ask yourself this question. Will foods consumed after 6 pm gain more calories than if they are eaten before 6 pm considering all other elements remain the same? For example, will 100 gm of brown rice contain more carbs in the night than in the morning? If you have a logical answer to this question, then worrying that eating late-night meals can increase fat reserves in your body is illogical.

The myth about eating late-night meals and becoming fatter could be based on the fact that many people tend to overeat during dinner than during daytime meals. From a metabolic perspective, there is no need not to eat food at a time that suits your needs, whether in the early morning or late at night. The food consumed in the morning is metabolized in the same way as the food consumed in the evening.

The problem only lies in the quantity of food consumed. If you can prevent overeating at night, and ensure you are always in a caloric deficit, then your intermittent fasting will achieve success no matter when you have consumed your meals.

How to Prevent Overeating

Now, that you know there is no scientific basis for the timing of your meals, you only must watch the quantity of food you eat during the eating window. Here are some tips to prevent overeating at any meal:

Take Away All Distractions

Eating while being distracted by the television, mobile devices, or even work is a common affliction of the modern times. Although this habit appears harmless, it is one of the most important causes of overeating. Studies have revealed that being distracted while eating tend people to consume more food than required. Turn off distractions such as phones, TVs, computers, etc. while eating so that you can focus on your meal. Paying attention to your food prevents binge-eating and makes eat be more conscious of 'feeling full' when your stomach is sufficiently fed.

Know Your Food Weaknesses

Identifying your food weaknesses and preparing for them can help you prevent overeating. For example, if you enjoy a bowl of ice-cream at night, make sure you don't stock it in your fridge. Prepare some healthy snacks and keep them ready when you want to have a treat during your eating window.

Also, keep all unhealthy snacks such as chips, cookies, and candies out of sight, or even better, don't keep any stock in your kitchen. Therefore, identify your weaknesses for unhealthy snacks, and keep them out of reach while keeping healthy options handy and accessible.

Cut Yourself Some Slack Occasionally

Restricting your intake excessively can make you feel deprived, and drive you to binge when you reach your limits. While meals based on whole, unprocessed grains are the best options, do make room for some indulgence sometimes.

You don't need to give up pizzas, chips, ice-creams, chocolates, etc. always. Occasionally treat yourself to a small piece of your favorite food so that your diet expectations are realistic and sensible. Just focus on whole-grained, unprocessed foods while giving yourself some flexibility to break the rules on special occasions. Avoid excessive and unrealistic restrictions.

Try the Volumetrics Method of Eating

Volumetrics is a method of eating in which you fill your plate with high-fiber, low-calorie foods such as non-starch veggies. In fact, when you start your eating window, let your first meal be a salad made with low-calorie vegetables including from the cabbage family followed with a drink of water. Give yourself about an hour, and then sit down to your full meal consisting of all three macronutrients. This approach is a great way to prevent binge-eating.

Don't Eat Directly from Containers

Eating ice-cream straight out of a carton, consuming takeouts directly from the box or eating chips from the packet, invariably make you overeat. Instead, serve out the food as portions on to your plate which will help you control calorie intake. Use measuring devices to find out the right portion sizes to meet your daily calorie requirement. Remember the point of an intermittent fasting eating method is to be in caloric deficit. Counting calories does matter to an extent.

Reduce Stress in Your Life

Excessive stress is one of the main reasons for binge-eating for most people in the modern world. Chronic stress increases the level of cortisol which is a hormone that enhances appetite driving you to eat more than needed. Consider using yoga, tai chi, mindful breathing, indulging in a favorite hobby, or any other activity that helps you reduce stress in your life. You will be able to control your calorie intake in a much better way by leading a stress-free life.

Eat Your Meals Mindfully

Focusing your entire body and mind on the moment of eating is called mindful eating. Your emotions, your thoughts, and your senses should all be converged in the act of eating your meal. For every bite, feel the texture of the food, recognize the flavors and smells, and focus on the chewing movements of your jaws.

Eat in small bites, chew thoroughly (in fact, counting to 20 for every bite works to keep your chewing thorough), and appreciate your food. Make mindful eating a habit in your life. Studies have revealed that eating mindfully reduces behaviors of binge-eating.

Include Plenty of Fiber-Rich Foods

There are studies which prove that consuming fiber-rich foods help you remain satiated for a long time. For example, if you were to eat fiber-rich oats for breakfast, then you will not feel excessively hungry during lunchtime reducing your food intake. Add beans to your salad, snack on nuts, and make sure every meal has a few veggies in it. Your fiber requirements will be sufficient met and you will feel fuller and less indulgent to overeat.

Maintain a Food Journal

This will help you get a tangible feel on the number of calories you are consuming. The food journal is a clear-cut unambiguous method of knowing exactly how much you ate at every meal. A food journal keeps you alert at all times. You will be very careful about what you eat because you are conscious that your actions are being recorded.

Moreover, studying this journal will help you understand when and why you tend to overeat which can help in preparing you to resist such temptations and situations. Studies have also shown that tracking your food intake helps in preventing overeating.

Eat With Like-Minded People

Food choices of your eating companions are bound to have an effect on your choices. Multiple studies prove that our food choices at each meal are influenced by how the other people at the table are eating. You will eat similar quality and quantity of food as your dining companions. If they order unhealthy food, so will you; and if they order healthy food, you will also follow suit. Try to eat with people who do not overeat.

Include A Lot More Proteins in Your Meals

Proteins keep you satiated for a longer time and also helps you prevent overeating at the next meal. Proteins help you stave off hunger pangs and cravings. Include Greek yogurt, nuts, and beans in your meals to prevent binge-eating.

Eat Very Slowly

Take your time over your meal. Don't rush through the activity because eating fast makes you overeat. Eating slowly helps you feel fuller with small portions and also reduces hunger. Eating slowly by chewing your food thoroughly can be an excellent way to prevent overeating. In fact, slow eating is directly connected to mindful eating.

Substitute Juices or Sugary Liquids with Water

Every time you feel thirsty, and reach out for juices or any sugary beverages, stop for a moment and think. That instant of a thought is enough to take your hand away from the bottle of soda or any sweetened drink and reach out for your water bottle instead.

Keep a bottle of water handy always. Keep sugary liquids and juices either out of your kitchen completely, or at least, out of easy reach, especially at a meal. There are studies which reveal that people who drank sweetened juices eat a lot more food at the meal than the people who drank only water.

Therefore, at every meal, be conscious and mindful of what and how you eat and drink to prevent overeating.

Conclusion

If you are the kind of person who can manage hunger pangs fairly easily, and is willing to wait a little while before indulging in a wholesome meal, and know and understand that you will not die from starvation if you simply extend your fasting period, then intermittent fasting can become second nature to you quickly and effectively. For others, it just needs a bit of working around the various challenges and temporary setbacks.

It might make sense to end on a positive note by giving you a brief summary of the benefits of intermittent fasting. So, here goes:

Flips the metabolic switch – Intermittent fasting reduces insulin spikes and compels your body to delve into its fast reserves to draw energy instead of depending on the glucose obtained from frequently consumed foods. The metabolism of your body switches from using glucose as the primary source of fuel to using fatty acids as the primary source of fuel, resulting in weight loss, and a healthy lifestyle.

Decreases visceral fat – Commonly referred to as belly fat, visceral fat is typically the first fat reserve target during intermittent fasting. Our body achieves increased health by using up the fat reserves from the belly fat.

Improved lipid profile – The using up of excessive fat results in a lot of good cholesterol being generated in place of bad cholesterol improving our overall lipid profile. An improved lipid profile translates to decreased risks of many health disorders including vascular and heart diseases.

Increases energy levels – Fats give 9 calories of energy per gm and glucose gives only 4 calories per gm. Switching the metabolic switch from glucose to fat, therefore, increases the energy released in our body.

Reduced oxidative stress and inflammation – The decreasing levels of fat tissues and leptin hormones from intermittent fasting reduces tissues inflammation and oxidative stress. Reduced inflammation results in reduced risks of diabetes and other health disorders.

Improved levels of the growth hormone – Intermittent fasting triggers increased production and release of the growth hormone essential for repair and regeneration. Increased levels of growth hormone also promote increased energy levels, lean muscle mass, and improved physical performance.

Intermittent Fasting is not a crash diet. It is a life-changing habit that can do wonders for your weight loss and healthy living goals. Before it becomes a deeply ingrained habit, you will encounter challenges and make mistakes as you go through the learning curve. It is important to take care of consuming sufficient calories that RETAIN muscle but USE up fat reserves. Getting everything perfect is going to take time, and a patient, committed approach is essential to make a success of your intermittent fasting journey.

Thank You!

Before you go, we would like to thank you for purchasing a copy of our book. Out of the dozens of books you could have picked over ours, you decided to go with this one and for that we are very grateful.

We hope you enjoyed reading it as much as we enjoyed writing it! We hope you found it very informative.

We would like to ask you for a small favor. <u>Could you please take a moment to leave a review for this book on Amazon?</u>

Your feedback will help us continue to write more books and release new content in the future!

66601700R00102

Made in the USA
Middletown, DE
06 September 2019